Guided Tour

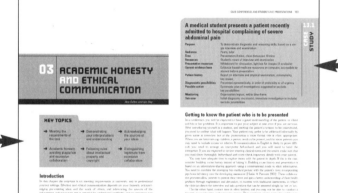

Case Studies

Case Studies illustrate
and expand on some
of the crucial ideas
and activities
explained in the book.

Key topics

Each chapter begins
with a Key Topics
panel that outlines the
major areas covered
in the chapter.

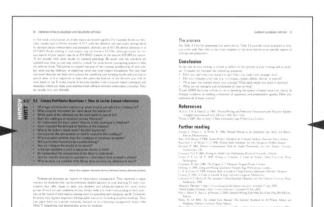

Handy Hints

Handy Hints through-
out the book highlight
key points and
provide tips on how
to communicate
effectively in
academic and
professional settings.

References and
Further Reading

At the end of
each chapter is a
References list for
the chapters and
a Further Reading
list covering books,
articles, and websites.

14.99 g
11.7.05

COMMUNICATING
IN THE HEALTH AND
SOCIAL SCIENCES

| Joy Higgs | Ann Sefton | Annette Street | Lindy McAllister | Iain Hay |

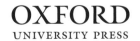

OXFORD
UNIVERSITY PRESS

OXFORD
UNIVERSITY PRESS

253 Normanby Road, South Melbourne, Victoria 3205, Australia

Oxford University Press is a department of the University of Oxford.
It furthers the University's objective of excellence in research, scholarship,
and education by publishing worldwide in

Oxford New York

Auckland Bangkok Buenos Aires Cape Town Chennai
Dar es Salaam Delhi Hong Kong Istanbul Karachi Kolkata
Kuala Lumpur Madrid Melbourne Mexico City Mumbai Nairobi
São Paulo Shanghai Taipei Tokyo Toronto

OXFORD is a trade mark of Oxford University Press
in the UK and in certain other countries

National Library of Australia
Cataloguing-in-Publication data:

Communicating in the health and social sciences.

Bibliography.
Includes index.
For undergraduates.
ISBN 0 19 551698 2.

1. Communication—Textbooks. 2. Communication in the social sciences—Textbooks.
3. Communication in medicine—Textbooks. I. Higgs, Joy.

808

Typeset by OUPANZS
Printed by Bookpac Production Services, Singapore

Contents

List of Figures   viii

List of Tables   ix

Contributors   xi

Preface   xiii

Acknowledgments   xiv

Part 1
Introduction

01 Communicating in the Health and Social Sciences   3
Joy Higgs, Lindy McAllister, and Ann Sefton

Part 2
Communicating in Academic and Fieldwork Settings

02 Study Skills   15
Iain Hay and Ann Sefton

03 Academic Honesty and Ethical Communication   22
Ann Sefton and Iain Hay

04 Learning Academic Writing   29
Joy Higgs, Lindy McAllister, and Joan Rosenthal

05 Learning to Write Essays and Assignments   42
Iain Hay and Lindy McAllister

**06 Searching the Literature and Managing the Collected
Data**   52
Ann Sefton and Annette Street

07 Referencing and Managing References   61
Joy Higgs, Joan Rosenthal, and Ann Sefton

08 Writing Journal Papers   73
Annette Street and Joy Higgs

09 Writing Theses   80
Joy Higgs and Annette Street

10 **Electronic Communication and Communicating in Flexible Learning**   90
Mary Jane Mahony

11 **Communicating in Problem-based Learning Classes**   99
Ann Sefton

12 **Writing Records, Reports and Referrals in Professional Practice**   105
Lindy McAllister, Iain Hay, and Annette Street

13 **Case Conferences and Student Case Presentations**   120
Ann Sefton and Annette Street

14 **Preparing a Community Health Proposal**   126
Lindy McAllister and Lucie Shanahan

15 **Communicating with the Community about Health**   137
Linda Portsmouth

Part 3

Presentation Styles, Skills, and Strategies

16 **Text Style and Formatting: Using Styles and Templates**   155
Charles Higgs and Joy Higgs

17 **Preparing Graphics and Tables**   161
Charles Higgs and Joy Higgs

18 **Preparing Posters**   169
Iain Hay and Ann Sefton

19 **Giving Talks in Class**   176
Annette Street, Iain Hay, and Ann Sefton

20 **PowerPoint Presentations**   184
Charles Higgs and Joy Higgs

21 **Presenting Talks at Conferences**   194
Annette Street and Iain Hay

Part 4

Interpersonal Communication

22 **Leading Groups and Meetings**   205
Joy Higgs and Mary Jane Mahony

23 **Talking with Colleagues, Patients, Clients, and Carers**   218
Lindy McAllister and Annette Street

24 **Working with Groups: Consulting, Advocating, Mediating, and Negotiating**   230
Ann Sefton and Lyndall Trevena

25 **Intercultural Communication**   239
Lindy McAllister and Annette Street

26 **Giving Feedback**   247
Lindy McAllister

27 **Learning to Communicate Clinical Reasoning**   254
Joy Higgs and Lindy McAllister

28 **Working as a Member of a Community Health Team**   260
Linda Portsmouth

Index   271

List of Figures

Figure 1.1	Issues in communication in the health and social sciences	5
Figure 1.2	A linear communication model	8
Figure 1.3	A transactional model of communication	9
Figure 6.1	Common fields in bibliographic databases	56
Figure 6.2	Example of a literature search audit table	57
Figure 7.1	Writing and inserting references by highlighting, cutting, and pasting: An example	69
Figure 10.1	What your flexible learning environment may include	92
Figure 11.1	Conceptual model of the PBL process	102
Figure 12.1	Example of a nurse's entry in a patient chart	110
Figure 15.1	The health communication process	138
Figure 16.1	Text sizes: Examples	157
Figure 17.1	Example of a bar chart: Pre-test and post-test scores for groups A–D	162
Figure 17.2	Example of a line graph: Test scores on VEM at hourly intervals	163
Figure 17.3	Example of a pie chart: Incidence of condition X per 10,000 population in Australian states and territories as percentage of total incidence	164
Figure 17.4	Clip art	166
Figure 17.5	Factors influencing health in the elderly	166
Figure 17.6	Images of health care	167
Figure 18.1	Two forms of poster layout	171
Figure 18.2	Poster example	174
Figure 20.1	Slide template and dot point layout	187
Figure 20.2	Picture as background	187
Figure 20.3	Slide with photograph	189
Figure 20.4	Slide with flowchart	189
Figure 20.5	Slide with graph	190
Figure 20.6	Slide with table	190
Figure 20.7	Editing a photograph	191
Figure 21.1	Example of an outline visual	198
Figure 22.1	Patterns of communication in groups	212
Figure 22.2	Simple action plan or meeting notes	213
Figure 22.3	Steps in problem solving	214
Figure 24.1	Common pathways for advocacy in health care and social services	233
Figure 24.2	Complex conflict situations	235
Figure 24.3	Negotiation involving a patient/client and multiple practitioners	236
Figure 24.4	Complex negotiation situation	237
Figure 27.1	Hypothetico–deductive reasoning	255

List of Tables

Table 1.1	Examples of factors influencing perception	9
Table 2.1	Catriona's time management framework	17
Table 4.1	Writing problems in order of importance and ways of addressing them	31
Table 4.2	Some basic rules of grammar	33
Table 4.3	The 10 P's of academic writing	34
Table 4.4	Technical aspects of writing	38
Table 5.1	Types of illustrative material and their labels	48
Table 9.1	Length of theses (guidelines only)	81
Table 9.2	Research paradigms	82
Table 9.3	Thesis structure	83
Table 9.4	Layout and presentation of theses	84
Table 9.5	Proposed headings for thesis	85
Table 10.1	Comparing asynchronous and synchronous communication	93
Table 12.1	Types of clinical reports in health professions	107
Table 12.2	Key strategies in report writing	116
Table 13.1	Preparing a case presentation	122
Table 14.1	Fields and locations of information to be included in a community profile	128
Table 14.2	Types of, constraints on, and ways to measure community needs	129
Table 15.1	Summary of health communication channels, communication activities, and media tools	141
Table 16.1	Justification of text	157
Table 17.1	Data for line graph	163
Table 17.2	Data for pie chart: States' incidence of condition X per 10,000 population	163
Table 17.3	Theories of benchmarking: Example 1	164
Table 17.4	Theories of benchmarking: Example 2	165
Table 17.5	Scores on three tests of men's and women's attitude towards child-rearing	165
Table 18.1	Fonts for posters	173
Table 18.2	Some connotations of colour	174
Table 19.1	Forms of presentation	177
Table 19.2	Advantages and disadvantages of various visual aids	180
Table 21.1	Structuring a presentation	198
Table 21.2	The use of different visuals	199
Table 22.1	Examples of group norms	207
Table 22.2	Roles of group members	208
Table 22.3	Leadership style and control	210

Table 23.1	Purposes of talk between professionals and colleagues, patients, and carers	219
Table 23.2	Outline of the ACT's Public Hospital Patients' Charter	220
Table 25.1	Some aspects of body language that vary across cultures	241
Table 25.2	Categories of intercultural communication skills	243
Table 26.1	Examples of reasons for giving feedback	249

Contributors

Professor Joy Higgs PhD, MPHEd, GradDipPhty, BSc
Faculty of Health Sciences
The University of Sydney

Emeritus Professor Ann Sefton PhD, DSc, MB, BS, BSc(Med)
formerly Faculties of Medicine and Dentistry
Deputy Chancellor
The University of Sydney

Professor Annette Street PhD, BEd(Hons)
Director, Latrobe/Austin Health Clinical School of Nursing
La Trobe University

Associate Professor Lindy McAllister PhD, MA(SpPath), BSpThy
School of Community Health
Charles Sturt University

Professor Iain Hay PhD, MA, GradCertTertEd, BSc(Hons)
School of Geography, Population and Environmental Management
Flinders University

Mr Charles Higgs MAppSci(SocEcol), MEd (ITET), GradDipEd(Tech), BSurv
Key Performance Consulting, Wollongong
Associate, Centre for Professional Education Advancement
Faculty of Health Sciences
The University of Sydney

Joan Rosenthal MA, BA, LACST
Centre for Professional Education Advancement
Faculty of Health Sciences
The University of Sydney

Linda Portsmouth MHlthComm, PGradDipHlthProm, BA, BAppSci
School of Public Health
Curtin University of Technology

Dr Mary Jane Mahony PhD, MS, GradDipDistEd, DipEd, BS
Director, Education Connections
Faculty of Health Sciences
The University of Sydney

Lucie Shanahan PostGradDipRuralHlth, BSpPath
South West Brain Injury Rehabilitation Service
Greater Murray Area Health Service, Albury

Dr Lyndal Trevena MPhilPH, MB, BS(Hons)
School of Public Health
Faculty of Medicine
The University of Sydney

Preface

Communicating effectively and considerately is a fundamental aspect of health care and of the many human interactions associated with providing professional services to people and communities. Its importance can often be neglected or taken for granted, because it seems so basic and 'everyday'. But when communication is poor the quality of health care and the collaborative relationships between people can suffer greatly. Similarly, in the education of health and social science professionals, communicating well is vital to the success of teaching and learning.

In this book we explore the nature of communication and the communication issues facing teachers, students, and professionals in the health and social sciences in their many tasks of communicating, from talking with patients and clients to giving talks at conferences and writing essays and theses. To include students from these professional groups, the book provides a number of chapters that are applicable across the groups, and have collectively termed the audience 'students preparing for entry to human service professions'. Some chapters are geared more to people working in clinical practice, others to those working in community and human services areas.

The book contains many discrete but interconnected peer-reviewed chapters, so that the tasks and challenges of communicating can be examined and practised in manageable 'chunks' but can also be linked to related tasks and to the bigger picture of why and how communicating well is important in the lives of human services professionals.

Joy Higgs and Ann Sefton

Acknowledgments

The collaboration and expertise of all of the authors of the book is acknowledged and appreciated. In addition we wish to particularly thank Joan Rosenthal, who, in addition to being one of the authors, provided valuable assistance in copy-editing. Our thanks also to Tim Campbell for his support of this process.

PART 1

INTRODUCTION

1   Communicating in the Health and Social Sciences   3

01 | COMMUNICATING IN THE HEALTH AND SOCIAL SCIENCES

Joy Higgs, Lindy McAllister, and Ann Sefton

KEY TOPICS

→ What are the health and social sciences?

→ What is communication?

→ What makes communication effective?

Introduction

This chapter provides a framework and introduction for the book. Here we discuss the nature and importance of communication in the health and social sciences. The term 'health and social sciences' refers to a variety of professional groups that provide social services and health-care services to people in community settings or in health-care facilities. These professions include medicine, dentistry, nursing, allied health (which includes a wide variety of professions such as physiotherapy, occupational therapy, radiography, speech pathology, and dietetics), psychology, social work, welfare studies, health education, and public health. We recognise that similar communication issues and tasks also face many professional groups in related social science disciplines and professions, such as economics, and in other professions, such as veterinary science.

Why is communication important in the health and social sciences?

Communication is the major tool used by health and social professionals to facilitate quality services for their clients. A client-centred approach to health and social services requires practitioners to understand clients' needs and desires for their health care and wellbeing and to communicate with clients and their families to develop shared goals and priorities. The effective teamwork that is required for efficient delivery of health-care services is based on good communication among team members. Sound communication skills are also essential to meet legal requirements related to documenting encounters, assessments, investigations, management plans, and treatment outcomes, and communicating these with relevant team members. Health and social professionals need to be proficient at communicating in a variety of communication styles and in a range of media (e.g. oral, written, and electronic forms). They need to continually monitor and develop their communication skills.

Communication

Communication is conferring through speech, writing, or nonverbal means (including body language) to create a shared meaning. It is considered to be a two-way process: that is, while talking, listening, writing, and reading can be one-sided, communicating involves two or more people sharing information.

To say that you have communicated means that a message has passed between you and another person or persons. Communication is effective when what people intended to say has been heard and the people involved have reached a point of shared meaning. Effective communication (whether oral or textual) requires:

- an intention to share information
- a desire to reach common understanding
- active listening (or reading) by the receiver
- an understanding by both parties of the person they are communicating with (including relevant aspects of background and culture)
- a commitment by the sender to use language that the receiver can understand and to communicate in a manner that is appropriate to the abilities and needs of the receiver (e.g. the client and family)
- a mutual willingness to understand the other person's point of view.

Issues in communication

Each professional is expected to attain competence in a range of discipline-specific and generic areas of performance. Throughout this book a number of key issues pertaining to these competencies are examined in relation to the practical aspects of helping health and social science students (and practitioners) to learn and use oral and written communication skills. These issues are shown in Figure 1.1 and are discussed in the following text.

Humanity

Communication, first and foremost, should be conducted in a spirit of humanity. As well as helping you provide high-quality professional services for individuals and the community, interpersonal skills are important in demonstrating respect for people, whether this is in the classroom or in professional practice.

Figure 1.1   Issues in communication in the health and social sciences

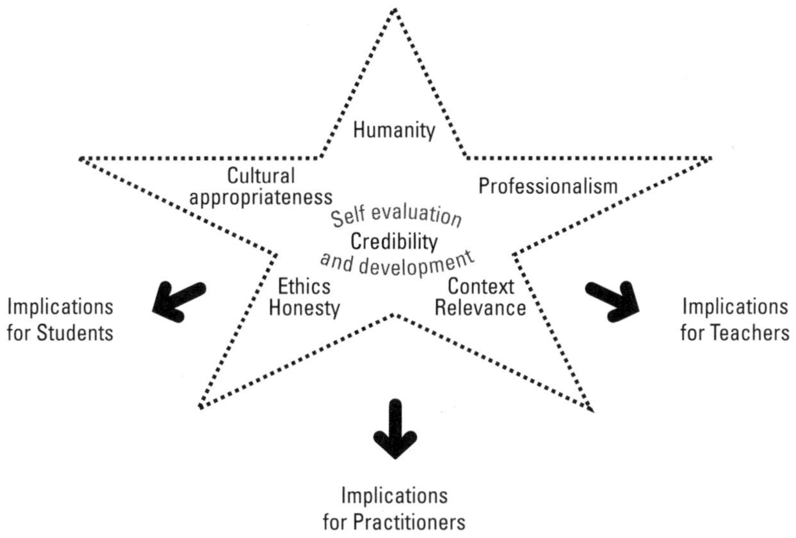

The relevance of context

Students are learners and neophyte professionals. They need to understand the context of each learning and professional practice task. What are the expectations of educators, patients, clients, and colleagues? More and more, the community expects health care and social services to be individualised, relevant, and timely. To achieve this, professionals must elicit information in order to understand and address their clients' needs. Listening carefully to clients is critically important. Moreover, students and professionals need to understand their audience to ensure that communication is appropriate. Different aspects of effective professional communication (e.g. formality of language, use of gestures or jargon, strategies for negotiation and conflict resolution) should be tailored to the audience.

Ethics and standards

Students and practitioners are bound by workplace and university rules and expectations that govern the performance of individuals and teams and indicate the conduct expected of them. These expectations can include 'unwritten rules', formal established ward protocols, and institutional regulations and expectations. Underpinning all of these workplace codes is the principle that health professionals are accountable for their practice. Members of different professions have codes of ethics that guide their behaviour. Related to ethical and workplace standards are the legal requirements of professional practice; written and oral communication must operate within requirements such as duty of care.

Academic/professional honesty

Chapter 3 highlights the issue of academic honesty as a central concern in professional studies. Academic honesty is particularly important in professional education, because the issues arising in student life are continued into professional practice, teaching, and research.

Professionalism

The notion of professionalism encompasses the issues of standards, codes of behaviour, and humanity, listed above, but also includes appropriate manners and styles of behaviour. Eraut (1994) portrayed professionalism as an ideology, characterised by the traits and features of an 'ideal type' profession. Relevant behaviours include showing respect for others, recognising the rights of others, demonstrating a duty of care, respecting the cultural backgrounds of others, and being responsible for the quality and appropriateness of one's practice and behaviour. Health and social science professionals are expected to demonstrate social responsibility (Prosser 1995), accountability, and a recognition of their limitations (Sultz et al. 1984). Professionalism in oral and written communications includes addressing the requirements of the task, demonstrating respect for individuals, meeting deadlines, and understanding best practice.

Cultural appropriateness

Professionals are expected to practise with integrity and personal tolerance, and to communicate effectively across language, cultural, and situational barriers (Josebury et al. 1990). Fitzgerald (2001, p. 153) defined 'culture' as 'the learned and shared patterns of perceiving and adapting or responding to the world characteristic of a society or population. Culture is reflected in such things as a society's learned, shared beliefs, values, attitudes and behaviours. Although culture is dynamic and ever changing, it maintains a sense of coherence.' 'Intercultural communication' refers to interactions between peoples of different cultures (Mullavey O'Byrne 1999). Such communication is a core part of interacting with people (patients, clients, colleagues, and carers) in the health and social sciences. Learning to be culturally competent in communication is an important goal of professional entry education.

Credibility

Whether people see you as a credible professional depends on how you address many of the issues above. Do people (fellow professionals as well as clients) think you demonstrate the professional practices and standards expected of your group? Are you responsive to your clients and colleagues? Do you consider and adapt to the age, background, and culture of the people with whom you are communicating? Do you keep good records? Your credibility as a professional will also depend on whether you can credibly justify your professional behaviour. Can you provide high-quality evidence to support your decisions? Do you keep your professional knowledge and skills up-to-date? Do you undertake research or evaluate the quality of your practice?

Self-reflection and self-evaluation

Finally, as a professional you need to reflect upon and critically evaluate your professional performance, your knowledge, and your skills. This evaluation also involves seeking feedback on your practice from supervisors, peers, and colleagues. Based on your self-evaluation, you can develop and implement strategies to improve your performance (for example, independently studying certain topics, practising skills you need to master, and participating in professional development activities). Developing the skill of honest self-evaluation as a student is an excellent preparation for professional life.

Types of communication

Communication can be formal or informal (Cats–Baril & Thompson 1997). Formal communication is often associated with systems and organisations in which information is distributed about the way the system operates (e.g. exam schedules, referral procedures, and institutional rules and regulations). People who receive such information use it to operate within that system (e.g. students read exam timetables and attend the right exams at the right time, and health professionals refer patients to the appropriate people). Such messages are explicit and 'official'. The presentation at conferences and in lectures of clinical and scientific work, generally supported by evidence, is also formal communication. The language of such communication can be called formal, scholarly, scientific, academic, professional, and so on.

Interestingly, much of what is called communication in organisations or via technology is simply the dissemination of information. Examples of dissemination media include the news media, mass electronic mailouts, and noticeboard bulletins. In these cases information is indeed sent. But has it been received? Have the sender and receiver reached a common understanding? Such questions cannot be answered in relation to one-way information flow. For this reason, we make a distinction between communication and the distribution of information.

Informal communication is comparatively spontaneous; it occurs in groups, among friends and colleagues, and between practitioners and their clients during professional interactions. The language used here is commonly more casual, informal, and colloquial. People talking informally, or sending notes, SMS texts (short messages via phone), or emails often use incomplete sentences, commonly understood language or jargon, abbreviations, and examples rather than detailed evidence. In communicating with patients or clients, practitioners usually need to 'de-jargon' their messages and should adapt their language to the client's circumstances (that is, take into account their client's language, culture, age, educational background, level of wellness, and comprehension). When we speak of effective or good interpersonal communication, we are mainly referring to informal communication that takes into consideration all the relevant circumstantial factors and addresses them effectively.

The communication process

The process and theory of communication has been discussed by many authors (e.g. Adler & Rodman 2003; Baker et al. 2002; Tyler et al. 2002). At the most simple level, textual or oral communication occurs between two people: a sender (source) and a receiver. A message is delivered through a channel (or more than one channel), a medium that connects the sender and the receiver. Feedback passes from receiver to sender. The process involves the sender encoding data to form a message and the receiver decoding the message. To encode, the sender translates the data or information he or she wants to communicate into a message that is appropriate in form and content for the purpose and audience. In decoding, the receiver may know, guess, or assume the purpose of the sender's message and may be influenced by personal perceptions, by background or intentions, by the medium of communication, or by interference (noise) associated with the message. The feedback the receiver gives to the sender may be verbal or nonverbal (e.g. nodding and smiling) and may include questions, evidence of understanding or of confusion, and emotions such as anger or pleasure. At this point the sender is actually receiving a message on how effective the communication has been, and needs to respond accordingly.

'Noise' can include distractions, perceptions, the language used, the type of message (e.g. good news or bad news), the appearance and body language of the people involved, and the type and style of feedback received, including the reply (e.g. a return SMS or email message). Possible channels of communication include verbal, written, electronic, and visual (including signs and body language) media. Each of these factors influences the effectiveness of communication. If you want to communicate effectively, you must consider the impact of each of these factors on the process and outcomes of communication.

Figure 1.2 A linear communication model

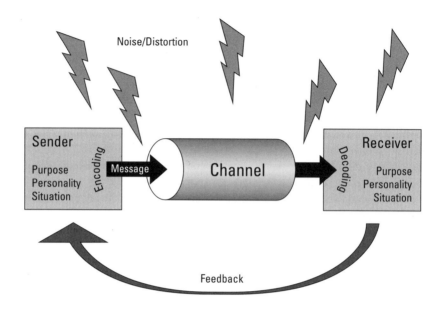

Figure 1.2 portrays the processes described above in a 'linear' model. Most communication, however, operates in a more complex or transactional manner (Adler & Rodman 2003; DeVito 2001; Tyler et al. 2002). Transactional communication involves:
- simultaneous sending and receiving of messages by two or more people.
- perception, which is 'the process by which we make sense of, and understand ourselves and others' (Tyler et al. 2002, p. 26). Perception involves selecting what we pay attention to from the mass of stimuli that impinge on our daily lives, and then organising and interpreting these stimuli to make sense of them. This interpretation is influenced by our existing knowledge, values, cultural background, and view of reality. Table 1.1 summarises a range of variables that influence perception.
- fluid rather than static communication; that is, communication is not an isolated act, but rather is part of a larger, complex set of interactions and relationships. Indeed, people themselves are constantly changing.
- relational rather than individual communication; that is, communication is something we do *with* other people not *to* them.
- a variety of communication channels (e.g. written, verbal, and electronic media).
- inevitability (i.e. we communicate even if we do not intend to), irreversibility (i.e. we cannot 'uncommunicate' something that has been communicated), and non-repeatability (i.e. the people and setting constantly change, so the precise circumstances cannot be repeated).
- filtering, modification, and interpretation of messages sent and received, based on the communicators' past experience and their frames of reference (e.g. values and cultural background).
- complex noise sources and patterns. As well as audible noises, such as traffic sounds and music, there are psychological noises and semantic noise. These terms refer to differences or difficulties in the way people use the symbols of language, especially words.

Table 1.1 Examples of factors influencing perception

Demographic factors (this is relatively accessible information)

• Physical location	• Past experience
• Culture	• Education
• Language	• Religion
• Gender	• Socio-economic position
• Age	• Occupational status

Psychographic factors (these variables are often less accessible)

• Assumptions	• Perspectives (points of view)
• Preconceived ideas	• Professional bias or disposition
• Biases and prejudices	• Personality
• Attitudes	• Expectations
• Values and beliefs	• Tastes and preferences (e.g. in fashion and music)
• Interests	• Past experiences
• Likes and dislikes	• Mood, motivation, etc

Source: Based on Tyler et al. 2002, p. 26

We must also recognise that the effectiveness of communication depends on the situation (the people involved and the physical, emotional, and task setting as well as the context and goals of the communication). Figure 1.3 presents this more complex transactional model of communication.

Figure 1.3 A transactional model of communication

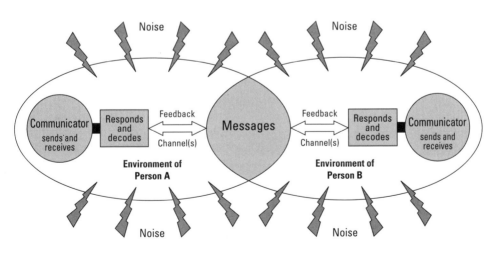

Source: Based on Adler & Rodman 2003; DeVito 2001; Tyler et al. 2002

Learning communication skills

In this section we consider some important communication skills that can be developed through practice.

Understanding the topic or message to be communicated

Being an effective communicator involves learning about the topic you want to communicate about and understanding it well, or at least better than you originally did. Sometimes this understanding comes during the communication process, as in a dialogue with others. Understanding the topic often means being able to look at it from multiple perspectives; for instance, looking at the pros and cons, and looking at the issue from different angles (say from the perspectives of cost–effectiveness and human interest).

Explaining well

Having understood your topic well, you must frame your message, identify the key points you need to explain, and communicate them clearly to your receiver(s). When you are trying to explain something it is often helpful to cover the following points: What do you want to communicate? Who is involved? Where and when is it occurring? How is it done or how does it work? Why does this happen? Why is it necessary or why should this happen?

In written communication, such as patients' notes, essays, and journal papers, explaining can take the form of clearly documenting the history or treatment, setting out the rationale for a proposed treatment regime, referring a patient to another professional, presenting an argument, or reporting on research. Such communication needs to be clear, relevant, and appropriate in length, content, and style. For example, medical prescriptions and requests for investigations need to be correct and unambiguous; and clinical notes need to contain clear and relevant information to facilitate communication between care providers and to meet legal and ethical standards.

Being person-centred

Being person-centred rather than task-centred involves using skills such as active listening or reading, empathic understanding, and cultural competence. The goal here is to genuinely hear and understand the sender's message and to acknowledge both the message and the person.

Active listening to oral communication and active reading of text (written or electronic) involves paying attention to the sender and to what he or she is trying to say or ask. It includes conveying interest, concern, and attention, and demonstrating that you want to hear what the person has to say. In face-to-face oral communication, body language plays a large part in showing interest. In other verbal communication (e.g. telephoning), interest can be shown by your tone of voice. In interactive text communication (e.g. SMS, email, and electronic bulletin boards) the style of language, the words used, and the order of content of your message can show how well you are attending to the other person's messages. For instance, you can show interest by acknowledging or commenting on the other person's message before sending your own.

Empathy is 'the ability to enter the perceptual world of the other person, to see the world as they see it. It also suggests an ability to convey this perception to the other person.' (Burnard 1997, p. 172). Empathy is not about feeling sorry for the other person, but about demonstrating a willingness to explore the other person's concerns and point of view, allowing and encouraging the other person to express themselves fully and to have their communication needs met. Fundamentally, health and social science professionals seek to foster the health and wellbeing of people and communities. This is achieved in part through supportive communication. Carlopio et al. (1997) detailed eight attributes of supportive communication, shown in Handy Hint 1.1.

1.1   Supportive communication principles

HANDY HINT

Supportive communication is:

- problem-oriented, not person-oriented; asking 'How can we solve this problem?'
- congruent, not incongruent; communicating real effects, not pretending; e.g. 'Your behaviour really upset me'
- descriptive, not evaluative; describing, not blaming or criticising; e.g. 'This is what I think happened and what I suggest we do'
- validating, not invalidating; e.g. 'I have some ideas, and I'd like to hear your suggestions too'
- specific, not global; e.g. 'You interrupted me three times just then' rather than 'You always take over the conversation'
- conjunctive, not disjunctive; relating your input to what is being discussed; e.g. 'In relation to that point, I'd like to suggest ...'
- owned, not disowned; e.g. 'I would like to pick up your idea about this case because ...'
- supportive listening, not one-way listening; e.g. 'What do you think would solve this problem?'

Source: Based on Carlopio et al. 1997, p. 224

Health professionals need to be competent in many areas of their practice. To be *culturally* competent requires going beyond token gestures in acknowledging another person's culture, beyond the use of stereotypical images and responses to cultural differences. Cultural competence involves seeking a clearer understanding of what it means to belong to the culture of the person with whom you are interacting, and adapting your manner of interaction as well as your professional services to that person's needs and background.

Self-monitoring

As with any complex skill, effective communication requires you to be aware of how and how well you are interacting with others. This involves learning to observe your own behaviour and its effects on other people, and developing strategies to see if others have understood your messages, as well as you understanding theirs. You could 'sum up' the key points made, check next steps or deadlines, or ask if the other person wants to add any points to the discussion. Being open to feedback from others is often a key to success in self-monitoring.

Being professional

In many parts of this book the issue of communicating professionally is addressed. Communicating professionally includes showing respect for people, providing sound evidence or arguments to support your proposed or actual actions, and working within the relevant ethical and legal parameters of professional health practice.

Conclusion

Professional communication in the health and social sciences is both challenging and rewarding. Effective communication is an essential aspect of sound practice. Communication competence involves being able to achieve your goals in communication and allowing others in the communication process to achieve theirs, as well as supporting and improving the relationship that frames the communication. Understanding and learning the skills of communication is an important part of your socialisation into the health professions. In the chapters that follow, many aspects of oral, embodied, written, and electronic communication are examined, along with guidelines and handy hints to help you become a competent communicator.

References

Adler, R. B. & Rodman, G. 2003, *Understanding Human Communication*, 8th edn, Oxford University Press, New York.

Baker, E., Barrett, M. & Roberts, L. 2002, *Working Communication*, John Wiley & Sons, Milton, Qld.

Burnard, P. 1997, *Effective Communication Skills for Health Professionals*, 2nd edn, Stanley Thornes, Cheltenham, UK.

Carlopio, J., Andrewartha, G. & Armstrong, H. 1997, *Developing Management Skills in Australia*, Longman, Melbourne.

Cats-Baril, W. & Thompson, R. 1997, *Information Technology and Management*, Irwin, Chicago.

DeVito, J. A. 2001, *Human Communication: The Basic Course*, 9th edn, Longman, New York.

Eraut, M. 1994, *Developing Professional Knowledge and Competence*, Falmer, London.

Fitzgerald, M. H. 2001, 'Gaining knowledge of culture during professional education', in *Practice Knowledge and Expertise in the Health Professions*, eds J. Higgs & A. Titchen, Butterworth-Heinemann, Oxford, pp. 149–56.

Josebury, H. E., Bax, N. D. S. & Hannay, D. R. 1990, 'Communication skills and clinical methods: A new introductory course', *Medical Education*, vol. 24, pp. 433–7.

Mullavey O'Byrne, C. 1999, 'Issues in intercultural and international learning in health science curricula', in *Educating Beginning Practitioners: Challenges for Health Professional Education*, eds J. Higgs & H. Edwards, Butterworth-Heinemann, Oxford, pp. 143–9.

Prosser, A. 1995, *Teaching and Learning Social Responsibility*, Higher Education Research and Development Society of Australasia, Canberra.

Sultz, H. A., Sawner, K. A. & Sherwin, F. S. 1984, 'Determining and maintaining competence: An obligation of allied health education', *Journal of Allied Health*, vol. 13, no. 4, pp. 272–9.

Tyler, S., Kossen, C. & Ryan, C. 2002, *Communication: A Foundation Course*, 2nd edition, Prentice Hall Australia, Sydney.

PART 2

COMMUNICATING IN ACADEMIC AND FIELDWORK SETTINGS

2	Study Skills	15
3	Academic Honesty and Ethical Communication	22
4	Learning Academic Writing	29
5	Learning to Write Essays and Assignments	42
6	Searching the Literature and Managing the Collected Data	52
7	Referencing and Managing References	61
8	Writing Journal Papers	73
9	Writing Theses	80
10	Electronic Communication and Communicating in Flexible Learning	90
11	Communicating in Problem-based Learning Classes	99
12	Writing Records, Reports, and Referrals in Professional Practice	105
13	Case Conferences and Student Case Presentations	120
14	Preparing a Community Health Proposal	126
15	Communicating with the Community about Health	137

02 STUDY SKILLS

Iain Hay and Ann Sefton

KEY TOPICS

Finding time for study:

→ Task assessment → Time assessment → Sticking to your timetable

→ Planning space for study → Getting even more organised → Getting involved

Introduction

Effective study skills are a foundation to learning success. This chapter sets out some vital elements of successful study. Many of the ideas outlined here, particularly those to do with effective time management, will serve you well in study as well as in the workplace. Probably the most important key to successful study at university (or anywhere, for that matter) is careful time and task management.

Finding time for study

Task assessment

At the beginning of each semester, teaching staff should provide you with a fairly clear indication of all class times, clinical placements, and assessment requirements. This will include details of due dates, assignment values, and so on. Plot all of the placements and assignment due dates on a calendar or year planner. You will probably find 'pile-ups' of assignments due just before and after the mid-semester break and a short time before exams commence at the end of the semester. To avoid the stresses of trying to complete all of these assignments at the same time, you will need to plan your work.

HANDY HINT ☞ **2.1 Planning is the key**

It is worth knowing before you start the semester that your lecturer will probably be rather unsympathetic to any claims that you could not do a particular assignment because of a clash of due dates. Most lecturers will argue that it is up to you to deal with that kind of problem by planning your work.

Look at your calendar of due dates and consider the work required to complete each piece of assessment. How much time do you think you need to finish each assignment? Be realistic. For instance, a good 2,000-word essay is going to take more like 2 weeks to write than 2 days. Think about the time you will need to find relevant references, gather material, read and take notes, and write, type, and edit. You might then consider doubling the amount of time you expect tasks will take to get a more accurate assessment of how long it really will take!

You have now completed the first part of a successful time-management plan. You know what tasks you have to complete and roughly how long they will take. The next part of the plan is to work out how much time you actually have to work on projects and exactly when you will work on them.

Time assessment

To know how much time you have and when you can complete tasks you will need to draw up a 7-day timetable broken into 1-hour intervals (see, for example, Table 2.1). What regular commitments do you have each week? For instance, you might have child-minding responsibilities, a part-time job three evenings a week, regular sports commitments on Saturdays and Thursdays, and so on. Record these on your timetable together with your lecture, clinical, and other class times to generate a diary template for your week. You can now use this as the basis for planning study and other activities for each day or week of the semester.

Table 2.1 shows you the time-planning skeleton created by full-time student Catriona, who, for this semester, has 8 hours of lectures each week, two 3-hour lab classes, and two 1-hour tutorials. Catriona also works on Thursday evenings and Saturday mornings at a local supermarket, and has two regular hockey commitments each week. As you may be aware, many students in the health and social professions also must complete a clinical-practice component lasting several weeks during the semester. If that were the case for Catriona, she would need to devise an additional time-management framework. It would need to take account of the different time and location arrangements associated with her clinical placement.

Table 2.1 Catriona's time management framework

	Mon.	Tues.	Wed.	Thurs.	Fri.	Sat.	Sun.
8.00 a.m.						Job at Coles	
9.00 a.m.		Tutorial	Lecture		Lab	Job at Coles	
10.00 a.m.	Lecture	Tutorial		Lecture	Lab	Job at Coles	
11.00 a.m.					Lab	Job at Coles	
12.00 p.m.		Lecture	Lecture			Job at Coles	
1.00 p.m.							
2.00 p.m.						Hockey game	
3.00 p.m.	Lecture		Lecture	Lab		Hockey game	
4.00 p.m.		Lecture		Lab		Hockey game	
5.00 p.m.				Lab			
6.00 p.m.							
7.00 p.m.			Hockey training	Job at Coles			
8.00 p.m.			Hockey training	Job at Coles			
9.00 p.m.				Job at Coles			
10.00 p.m.				Job at Coles			

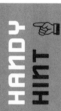

2.2 Using Excel for time management

Try creating your time management template in software such as MS-Excel. This offers the advantage of allowing you to use search functions to find specific events within your semester's timetable.

HANDY HINT

Catriona uses copies of this timetable to help organise her time for other activities during the week; for example, she can add details of social events and everyday tasks like shopping. But before she fills in the spaces on her timetable with these kinds of activity, there is the small matter of the semester assignment schedule to consider. It is in the times on the week-to-week diary not occupied by classes and other 'immovable' commitments that you, like Catriona, must take the opportunity to complete your assignments, read for classes, and so on.

Looking at the time-management framework, we can see that there are times of the week when large blocks of time are available and other times when there is only an hour or so available between fixed commitments. Catriona might consider dedicating her long blocks of time, like those on Monday, Thursday, and Friday, to working on big projects (e.g. writing essays and preparing for in-class talks) and using the shorter interludes (e.g. Tuesday 11–12 a.m.) for activities like reading articles, photocopying, and doing library searches. To some extent, the choices about what to do in each of the time slots will depend on where she is (at home or at university) as some tasks can only be done on campus.

Catriona now knows exactly how much time she has available each week to complete all her coursework tasks. She must now allocate an appropriate number of days to each assignment and then work out in which weeks (if not the precise days) of the semester she will work on each assignment, setting target dates for completion.

The following piece of news may be horrifying, but it is a useful rule of thumb: if you are enrolled as a full-time student you are generally expected to dedicate as much time to your studies as someone would devote to a full-time job (say 36–40 hours per week). Only a small part of study time will be taken up with formal class contact. For instance, Catriona has only 16 hours of classes each week. To complete all of the work in her course (essays, reports, etc.), she will probably need to study for an additional 20–25 hours each week. Like most people, Catriona might be inclined to avoid this in the first few weeks of semester, but that error would haunt her as the semester progressed! If you make your study time regular and constant throughout the entire semester, you will go a long way toward avoiding the need for panic-stricken 'cramming' at exam time and less-than-useful 2 a.m. essay-writing sessions the night before each paper is due. Note that a part-time student would spend proportionately less time studying. A half-time student might spend about 20 hours each week at lectures, reading, attending laboratories, and so on.

Leave a little extra time each week to cope with the unexpected. Things will happen that divert you. A friend from overseas may arrive unexpectedly; your oven could explode; or your housemate might have a family emergency to deal with. Anticipate the likelihood of such events by building in spare time in your diary. If you overfill your timetable you are likely to become frustrated that you cannot complete things.

Now that you have worked out your timetable, do you actually have enough time for study, work, and leisure? How much time do you have for study? Is it enough? Does anything need to be reorganised? Adjust your timetable until you believe you have sufficient time for study and those other activities you need to be involved in. If this does not work, you may need to reconsider some of your non-study commitments, amend your enrolment, or seek some assistance from a study counsellor.

HANDY HINT ☞ 2.3   Getting advice on time management

If you are putting together a time-management scheme for the first time, it may be helpful to visit a study counsellor with a draft of your timetable, even if you are happy with it, or to discuss your plan with a fellow student, just to ensure that you are giving adequate consideration to all your study and personal commitments.

Sticking to your timetable

The final and critical part of successful time management is sticking to the timetable you have so carefully created. Be sure to use allocated times for allocated tasks. Although you might find that some days seem unproductive and you cannot, for example, write any 'keepable' text for an essay, take comfort in knowing that such days are often times when you are incidentally consolidating ideas in your mind and they are often rewarded by highly productive days soon after.

Time management of the sort set out here may *seem* regimented and restrictive. But it allows you to exercise control over your work and study, rather than have it control you. A firm timetable may actually make you feel freer because you will know when you are relaxing that you have the right to do so. You will also feel a sense of achievement for having your work and study under control. In later employment, you will find that good time management skills developed during study will stand you in good stead.

Planning space for study

Now you have the time, you need to find the place: the second key to study success is territorial. Find a place that is pleasant, quiet, and well-lit, a place where you will be able to work relatively undisturbed. If you can, avoid working on the dining-room table or in front of television because, despite their other skills, 'Judge Judy' and your neighbours in Ramsey Street won't help you study. Try to make your study space (e.g. an office or part of your bedroom) somewhere dedicated to that task, because it helps if you are able to get up and walk away from your study for periods of rest and relaxation. If you cannot find an appropriate place at home you might be able to find a desk or carrel in the university library or in your local library, where you can work comfortably and without being bothered.

Getting even more organised

The third key to successful study is organisation. If you have good time management and task management skills, you will have gone a long way down this path. To capitalise on your skills in these areas, it is useful to be organised in other ways too. Of particular help is a good filing system—exciting, eh? Create a filing system that works for you. It must allow you to find all your lecture, workshop, and reference material quickly and to know that your notes are complete (i.e. no missing pages). You might find it helpful to keep your chronologically ordered lecture notes in a folder or filing cabinet. To these notes you can add relevant photocopies of articles and chapters. Alternatively, extra notes might be kept in another system, catalogued by author, for example. You might also find it helpful to use software such as EndNote, ProCite, and Reference Manager (see also Chapter 7). These reference-management tools allow you to record bibliographic and other details of material you have read and can also easily generate correctly formatted reference lists for essays and other written reports. Importantly, they will allow you very quickly to search all of the references you have read to help find key sources for different assignments.

2.4 Safeguarding your notes

Whenever you can, avoid carrying an entire semester's notes with you or leaving them in your car. Every year lecturers are presented with distraught students whose notes—and often the cars containing their notes—have been stolen.

HANDY HINT

Getting involved

The final important study skill is simply *getting involved in learning*. Succeeding at university is about teaching *and* learning. Academic staff (your lecturers, tutors, and laboratory demonstrators) do their best with the resources available to them to teach well. But the relationship does not stop there. A critical element behind your success is your engagement with learning. It is important that you take learning seriously and that you involve yourself in it. You can do this in a variety of ways.

First, study things you are interested in, not necessarily those things your friends and relatives say you 'should' enrol in.

Second, when you are in class, listen to understand. If there is something you do not follow, ask! It can sometimes be a little intimidating to put your hand up in a large lecture class, but take comfort in knowing that if you do not understand something there is a strong chance others do not too. If you are too shy to speak out in class, see the lecturer afterwards or send an email query to seek clarification. If you ask politely and are not unreasonable in your request, most lecturers and tutors will be willing to help.

Third, when you are reading books and articles, be sure you are reading to comprehend. Do not make the mistake of assuming that because you have marked a page with a highlighter that you have read it. It is often helpful, though sometimes difficult, to write yourself two or three sentences summarising the key points of an article or book. When you challenge your mind to encapsulate the message of a large work, you will know whether you have understood it. You might also find it beneficial to compare your summary with that of someone else in your class, or to discuss it with your lecturer/tutor to confirm your interpretation. The summaries you produce can also be useful additions to the notes you make about books and articles in reference-management software.

Fourth, consider working in an informal study group. Many students find that their learning is enhanced through discussion. Explaining your ideas to another person is particularly constructive, and other people can help you think about issues in new ways.

Fifth, keep good records. When you do literature searches, keep a record of the databases you have searched and the key words you used; keep the references you use in a logical filing system; take comprehensive and comprehensible notes, recording page numbers and all bibliographic details; ensure that photocopies are legible and include full bibliographic details; and so on (see Chapters 6 and 7 for more details). In the long run, these records will save you a great deal of time.

Conclusion

Intelligence, good communication skills, and innate flair for a subject are certainly helpful for success at university study, but good study skills are absolutely vital. If you wish to do well at university and do so with relatively little anguish, it is critical that you develop time-management skills, get organised, and get involved in your learning. You can also take heart in knowing that many of the time and organisational skills you practise and refine at university will hold you in good stead for any professional role you play.

Further reading

Aston University 2003, 'Time management' <http://www.aston.ac.uk/welfareservices/studyskills/time_management.htm> accessed 21 March 2003.

Hay, I., Bochner, D. & Dungey, C. 2002, *Making the Grade: A Guide to Successful Communication and Study*, Oxford University Press, Melbourne. (See especially Chapter 2.)

Marshall, L. & Rowland, F. 1998, *A Guide to Learning Independently*, 3rd edn, Open University Press, Maidenhead, Berks.

South-Western 2003, 'Time management' <http://www.swcollege.com/web_resources/bktimemg.htm> accessed 21 March 2003.

University of Victoria (Canada) 2003, 'Learning skills program' <http://www.coun.uvic.ca/learn/ timemgt.html> accessed 21 March 2003.

03 | ACADEMIC HONESTY AND ETHICAL COMMUNICATION

Ann Sefton and Iain Hay

KEY TOPICS

→ Meeting the requirements of the task

→ Demonstrating your interpretations and understanding

→ Acknowledging the sources of your ideas

→ Academic honesty: avoiding plagiarism and excessive collaboration

→ Following rules about intellectual property and copyright

→ Distinguishing legitimate from excessive collaboration

Introduction

In this chapter the emphasis is on meeting requirements at university and in professional practice settings. Effective and ethical communication depends on your honestly acknowledging pre-existing ideas and the work of others, and referencing the sources of the information and arguments; this is essential for professional credibility and an important part of your academic honesty. You also need to understand the limits of legitimate collaboration with your colleagues, both in individual and in group tasks.

Honesty and trust are fundamental requirements of everyone at university. Effective, professional practice is based on ethical values, and your obligations start when you are a student. You must respect the rights and sensitivities of both your fellow students and the clients or patients (and other relevant parties, such as carers and families) with whom you interact. You will be expected to accept responsibility for your actions, and to be truthful and open in all your activities. In practice situations, you will also be expected to meet the appropriate ethical standards within the professional discipline you are studying. By acting honestly and openly but sensitively at all times, you will ensure that you never disadvantage others.

General issues at university

Although educational and professional workplaces such as health-care institutions, schools, and community-service workplaces differ in their specific requirements, it is a general principle that you should not take advantage of fellow students, university staff, practitioners, clients, or patients you meet. Never take credit for work that is not yours. You will always be required to accept responsibility for your own actions, and to be honest and open in all your activities. You can expect others to behave similarly.

Universities and professional workplaces and their staff typically have expectations of students and practitioners, which they make clear through policies relating to matters such as ethical conduct, quality assurance, evaluation, and staff–student or patient–practitioner relationships. Not all breaches of ethical conduct are deliberate or seek advantage. In some cases, students transgress policies because they do not know how to find out what is expected of them. Nevertheless, by enrolling at your institution you are implicitly accepting the need to abide by its rules. While you are a student, it is up to you to read handbooks, guidelines, and policies to ensure that you understand the specific requirements. Ignorance is not an acceptable excuse for any failure to follow stated rules. Policies on standards of behaviour and ethics are usually found on a university's website (see examples listed in the Further Reading section at the end of this chapter). Individual faculties, departments, and practice settings may have particular expectations relating to honesty and ethical behaviour. It is your responsibility to read the specific guidelines and ensure that you understand what is expected, or to ask your teachers.

When the semester starts, ensure that you clearly identify your commitments. Plan so that you can attend all essential classes, contribute to group activities, complete individual assignments, and submit all your work on time. If your course is supported by Web-based resources, you might be able to catch up if you miss some non-compulsory contact time. Most students have jobs and/or family commitments, and staff usually understand such obligations. Special consideration may be given to students who are representing the university in some recognised activity. Nevertheless, you cannot expect to use your job, a social event, or a planned trip as an excuse for failing to meet a university obligation. If you anticipate difficulties in meeting a commitment, consult the relevant member of staff to determine what, if any, flexibility can be negotiated. If you have not already done so, you may need to revise your personal and employment schedule, rather than your university timetable.

Despite set requirements, universities generally allow for consideration to be given when students have difficulty in completing work on time because of illness or other adverse circumstances. If you find yourself in this position, you could, as well as following formal procedures to ask for special consideration, seek informal help from individual teachers, who might be sympathetic. However, most staff cannot allow excessive or repeated extensions of deadlines, because of their own commitments and because it is unfair to the students who complete tasks within the set time limit.

Self-care and recognising when you need help are crucially important for all students, and particularly those who are aiming to join professions in which good standards of behaviour and service to others are clear expectations. Should you become ill or experience a serious personal difficulty, don't hesitate to seek help (and the earlier the better). Notify the relevant faculty office or department or a key member of staff if the problem entails your absence from a required task (particularly an assessment) or if you will be away from your studies for longer than a few days. Find out what you can do to catch up and avoid penalties. Course and fieldwork supervisors or year, course, or subject coordinators are usually the appropriate people to approach. A faculty member may be assigned to assist students in difficulties (e.g. a Sub-dean or a Dean for Students). Most institutions require you to present a medical certificate for an illness lasting more than a few days. Find out what the requirements are. You may also need to provide other evidence if adverse circumstances have impeded your progress. You may need such evidence if you have a disability that requires some concessions (e.g. variation in examination conditions).

Overall, you need to be clear about what is expected of you. If you are uncertain, consult guidelines provided by the university, faculty, or department(s). Seek an appointment to clarify particular issues with a member of staff. *Never* rely on the student grapevine for accurate information about what is acceptable or appropriate; it is notoriously unreliable.

Academic honesty

Essentially, academic honestly serves to ensure that each student receives due credit for his or her own work. It is obviously unfair to copy from books or journals without proper acknowledgment of the source of the information, or to use another student's work, or to fail to contribute constructively to a group assessment. In order not to disadvantage fellow students and staff, you are expected to plan your work so that you can assist others in collaborative projects and so that you can meet essential deadlines, your own and those of the group. Seek help early if you are in difficulty or if you don't fully understand what is expected of you. Fulfilling requirements on time is essential in professional life. Most universities' websites provide institution-specific guidance on the meaning of academic dishonesty and plagiarism. Check your own university's site, and see the examples in this chapter.

Intellectual property

Another aspect of academic honesty relates to intellectual property, which is the 'research, words and ideas generated by an author' (see Baker et al. 2002, p.164). When a member of staff, a student, or a team makes an original discovery or offers a re-interpretation of ideas, it becomes the intellectual property of that individual or team. It is their right to publish the discovery or, through the university, to pursue the possibility of developing it and/or selling the rights, or patenting it. For further information see the Australian Government Intellectual Property website (listed in the Further Reading section at the end of the chapter).

Copyright

When an author's work is published, it becomes subject to copyright and may not be reproduced except with the author's permission. You can also copyright your own original unpublished work by adding your name and the copyright symbol (©) after the title. It is generally accepted that you may photocopy a journal paper, a key diagram, or small sections from a book for your own study. Copying large sections or several chapters, however, breaches copyright. If you want to include a published diagram or illustration in an essay or paper, you must acknowledge the source. Some universities expect you to redraw the material yourself (check the precise requirements of your own institution). See also the Australian Copyright Council website (listed under Further Reading).

Plagiarism

It is important that you understand what constitutes plagiarism (a form of academic dishonesty) within your institution. The penalties for deliberate plagiarism can be severe. Plagiarism is defined on the University of Sydney website as 'presenting another person's ideas, findings or work as one's own, or … copying or reproducing work without due acknowledgment of the source'. Thus, if you quote the work or ideas of others, you must acknowledge this source (i.e. cite the reference for the work, including the page number if you are referencing a direct quote, figure, model, etc.). Examples of plagiarism include presenting written work taken from a published source or the Internet without acknowledging the original author(s), and copying the work of another student. Academic staff familiar with the relevant literature can often identify plagiarism of published materials. There are now electronic tools, such as *EVE2* (Essay Verification Engine) and *Turnitin*, that make it easier to detect plagiarism.

In some cases plagiarism reflects a lack of understanding about the importance of acknowledging other people's work, or uncertainty about how to reference material correctly. If you are unsure of the correct way to reference, ask your teacher or look up a referencing source. At the least you can indicate that the relevant ideas are derived from someone else, for example by saying '(Smith 2004, lecture notes)' or '(Chen 2004, personal communication)'. In other cases students plagiarise because they are not confident about expressing themselves in their own words. These may be the reasons behind a habit of copying other people's work, but they are not adequate excuses. You need to take action to address the underlying problem. If you feel unsure about what is expected, or have difficulty expressing yourself, discuss your problem with a member of staff. Read or re-read Chapters 6 and 7 of this book. Early in your program, some teachers may offer you the chance to submit work and have it reviewed before finally handing it in. Take that opportunity. It offers invaluable, specific feedback. If you are not confident with academic writing, particularly if English is not your first language, refer to Chapter 4 and seek help from university support services to develop skills in expressing yourself. Such assistance will often improve your confidence and enhance your communication generally, with colleagues, staff, and patients.

Ethical research work

In many programs you will be encouraged to do some research; honesty and trust are central features of all research. Research findings are accepted when the data are accurate, critically analysed, and honestly reported. Conclusions must be carefully drawn on the basis of rigorous, trustworthy analysis and interpretation. Rigorous standards of honesty are expected regardless of the duration of the research and the research mode (for example, whether it is based on reviewing texts or Web-based material or conducting laboratory, practice, or community work).

Ethical group work

There are considerable benefits from learning cooperatively in academic and practice teams and groups. In general, the most effective learning in groups comes when all members participate actively and complete required tasks. When undertaking a group project, it is important that the group determine roles and responsibilities from the outset, but be prepared to be flexible. Honesty in group interactions is essential. You must be prepared to both offer and accept help, but never take advantage of other members. It is clearly unfair to the rest of the group if someone fails to turn up and contribute, or doesn't complete agreed tasks. If the group is not working well, confront the problems collectively and resolve them before the situation deteriorates.

CASE STUDY 3.1

Group project

Groups of five students are required to prepare and present a poster on an aspect of smoking and community health in six weeks. The following guidelines will help the groups achieve these goals collaboratively and fairly.

Brainstorming (immediately)

- What knowledge and skills do we have (e.g. access to specific information, skills in IT, data analysis, and design)?
- What is the most interesting aspect of the subject to research and present?
- Agree on a broad direction, an outline, and a method of presentation.
- Divide responsibilities, focusing first on gathering information and data.
- Set a realistic timetable for individual preparation and meetings.

Ongoing meetings

- Review the data elements as they are contributed.
- Modify the tasks in the light of experience.
- Agree on a broad framework and design after data are collected.
- Settle on a 'message', layout, and means of preparation.
- Assemble the elements and finalise them well before the deadline.

Assessment

- If group members are to be individually assessed, agree beforehand on the contributions of each.

Particular difficulties can arise in collaborative work when the group is assessed collectively and given a single mark or grade. Students who do not participate or contribute equitably are unfairly or dishonestly taking advantage of their colleagues. The group needs to discuss the issue openly. If lack of participation is due to personal or health-related difficulties, fellow students are usually tolerant and willing to help. If it represents an unwillingness or inability to cooperate, the group needs to confront the issue. If it persists, the problem may need to be discussed with staff.

Many students find it helpful to learn in an informal, self-selected group. It is, however, important to establish what is legitimate cooperation for tasks that will be individually assessed. As you prepare an assignment, it is time-efficient to share the collection of references, and informal discussion of interpretations can help clarify issues. Nevertheless, everyone must independently hand in their own ideas and conclusions. Work must not be copied or written jointly if the assignment is meant to be completed individually.

Honesty in assessment:
Exams and individual assignments

The marks for individual assignments and exams should reflect each student's knowledge and skills at the time. If students are dishonest, they may gain an unfair advantage, but, more seriously for the community, they may be certified as qualified when they have not reached the required academic or practice standards. Dishonest behaviour is of particular concern when students are preparing for ethical professional practice.

In exams, it is dishonest to copy from or communicate with another student. You must not bring unauthorised materials to the test or substitute for another candidate. It is wrong to gain prior access to non-public exam papers, or to complete a secure exam paper outside the exam room. For fieldwork exams, make sure that you understand the exact requirements. It is good practice to review recent exam papers (usually kept in the library) before the formal exam. Check before any clinical or fieldwork examination what the exam conditions will be (for instance, whether or not you will have access to your patient's previous notes or your client's past records).

Be aware of the likely consequences of dishonesty. Procedures and penalties for academic misconduct vary between universities. They may also differ depending on the nature of the breach and the stage of development of the student concerned. Some universities may take into account particular circumstances, but others allow little latitude. Penalties range from a warning or cancellation of marks on an assignment to a fail in the unit of study or in the year or, at worst, expulsion. Understand your rights and responsibilities: you may be allowed to have support at any meetings in which your case is heard. If, for some reason, you feel that you have been treated unfairly, find out how you can appeal.

Students who know or suspect that a fellow student is behaving dishonestly are often unsure what they should do about it. University policy documents rarely offer any guidance on this issue. The culture generally discourages 'dobbing in' of fellow students, even though their misbehaviour disadvantages the rest of the class. Even if you have no more than a reasonable suspicion, you (perhaps with colleagues) can speak directly to the student concerned and it may prevent future occurrences. You may need to bring the matter confidentially to the attention of a member of staff, who might be in a better position to determine whether some dishonesty has occurred and to act on it.

Issues in clinical or fieldwork settings

As a student in the health or social sciences, you will be expected to meet the ethical standards of your professional group. You will be put into positions of trust by patients, clients, supervisors, and colleagues. You must respect confidentiality. You should be aware of local rules governing the interviewing of children and adolescents and those who may need a carer or interpreter to be present. Be aware of differences in values, beliefs, and attitudes, and respect your patients' or clients' views. You will also need to continually reflect on your practices and behaviours. As part of your ongoing development of sensitive and professional communication skills, you may find it useful to think critically and frequently about the following issues:

- Are you behaving in ways that you, the patient/client, and the broader communities of which you are a part believe to be morally right?
- Are you helping or potentially harming your patient/client?
- Are you demonstrating respect for your patient/client, colleagues, and staff?
- Are you meeting the prescribed expectations of professional relationships?
- Are you respecting your patient's/client's autonomy (their right to be regarded as an independent, self-determining individual)?
- Do you reflect after each encounter on the effectiveness of the communication?

If you work through the principles covered in the six questions set out here, you will have gone a long way toward ensuring that you and your patient or client have rewarding, mutually respectful meetings. These principles should assist you when you are asked to respect confidentiality and when you must ensure that you obtain informed consent to interviews, examinations, or treatments. If you become aware of a difficult issue or conflict, seek advice from your clinical or fieldwork educator or the relevant senior practitioner.

Maintaining honest and open communication is essential, but some dilemmas will inevitably confront you. Always be sensitive to people who have different needs and preferences. Be prepared in advance with an answer for any patient who demands a diagnosis or prognosis from you, or who is unhelpful or dismissive. Think how you might deal with the situation if a patient or client asks you not to reveal important information to other colleagues or team members. Outside of formal clinical or fieldwork presentations, you must protect the anonymity of your patients/clients by not disclosing information that would identify them personally.

Conclusion

All professions within the fields of health and social sciences demand consistently honest and ethical behaviour of practitioners. It is important to develop, demonstrate, and refine the high standards you will require in practice while you are a student. You should make sure that you understand the expectations that your university and future profession hold regarding honesty, but you must also be aware that it is *you* who is ultimately responsible for your ethical behaviour.

Further reading

Baker, E., Barrett, M. & Roberts, L. 2002, *Working Communication*, John Wiley & Sons, Milton, Qld.
Flinders University 2003, 'Academic dishonesty' <http://www.flinders.edu.au/studentinfo/acad_dishon.htm> accessed 21 March 2004.
O'Shea, R. P. 2002, *Writing for Psychology*, 4th edn, Thomson Learning, Melbourne.
University of Melbourne 2003, 'Academic honesty and plagiarism' <http://www.services.unimelb.edu.au/plagiarism/> accessed 2 April 2004.
University of Sydney 2003, 'Academic honesty in coursework' <http://www.chs.usyd.edu.au/PG/honesty.html> (search term 'honesty') accessed 21 March 2004.
University of Western Australia 2003, 'Cheating and other academic dishonesty' <http://handbooks.uwa.edu.au/undergraduate/poliproc/policies/Dishonesty> accessed 21 March 2004.
Trent Focus UK <http://www.trentfocus.org.uk/Resources/ethical_considerations_research.htm> accessed 21 March 2004.

Copyright

Australian Copyright Council website <http://www.copyright.org.au/> accessed 2 April 2004.
Australian Government Intellectual Property website <http://www.ipaustralia.gov.au/> accessed 2 April 2004.
CaNexus.com. 2004, *EVE2: Essay Verification Engine* <http://www.canexus.com/eve/abouteve.shtml> accessed 17 March 2004.
TURNITIN website <http://www.plagiarism.org/> accessed 2 April 2004.
WhatisCopyright.org 2004, 'What is copyright protection?' <http://www.whatiscopyright.org/> accessed 2 April 2004.

04 | LEARNING ACADEMIC WRITING

Joy Higgs, Lindy McAllister, and Joan Rosenthal

KEY TOPICS

→ What is scholarly or academic writing?

→ What are the purposes of academic writing?

→ What are the characteristics of academic writing?

→ Learning to write

→ Knowing what makes good writing

Introduction

Academic or scholarly writing is of particular importance to students and professionals in the health and social sciences. Writing is an important skill for a range of reasons: it allows you to communicate your knowledge to lecturers and members of the public; it helps you obtain satisfactory results in the classroom and practical settings; and it enhances your credibility as an emerging professional.

Students enrolled in tertiary education programs need to learn many skills of professional communication. One of these skills is being able to write in an academic or scholarly style.

This type of writing is used when writing essays, assignments, journal papers, research reports, and theses. Academic writing is a genre. It differs from the more colloquial language of a letter or a magazine article, the more colourful language and discursive style of a novel, and the more abbreviated style of lecture notes.

Characteristics of academic writing

Conventions of the academic writing genre include writing grammatically and clearly, punctuating according to the format required, using words precisely, avoiding long complex sentences, being consistent (with spelling, past/present/future tense, style, active/passive voice, etc.), explaining and minimising jargon, limiting slang and colloquial language, and avoiding ambiguity. The level of formality of your writing will vary with your audience. Following these conventions will help you get your message across in a manner that makes absorbing it as easy as possible for your readers. If your readers have to struggle and reread passages in order to make sense of your writing, it detracts from their appreciation of what you are saying. Readers should be able simply to focus on your message.

In addition to being clear, academic writing needs to present a credible case or position; hence, you must provide supportive evidence and arguments (and clear acknowledgment of the source(s) of your ideas and data). Academic writing also needs to be analytical and critical; your role is to critique, not blindly accept, data, opinion, research results, etc., in order to present a reasoned case. In Chapter 3 the ethical aspects of academic writing are discussed.

Writing types and formats

As a professional in the health or social sciences you will use different types of professional writing: essays, journal articles, project reports, case notes, management plans, and many more. Each of these types of writing has a typical format or structure, which may be particular to your profession, your workplace, or even your team or ward in the case of client reports and records. Most universities produce a guide to written assignments, which provides essential advice. If you are not sure of the format to use for a particular piece of writing, or if there seems to be no specific required format, ask your lecturer or fieldwork educator for a good example of the type of writing required. You can also refer to other chapters of this book for advice on structuring essays, assignments, reports, clinical/fieldwork records and referrals, journal articles, and theses (i.e. reports of research degree studies).

Different types of writing serve different purposes. For example, essays typically argue, defend, or critique a point of view. A thesis develops and provides evidence and support for a position. Fieldwork reports primarily inform patients/clients or colleagues about the nature of a patient's or a population's needs and problems, and about recommendations for intervention. File notes inform others involved in case management about your treatment of a client to date, and also provide a record of the amount, timing, and nature of service. Community proposals may include a needs assessment, program proposal, budget, and plan for evaluation. Referrals for assessment or treatment by other professionals or colleagues are requests for an opinion or service. A case presentation informs colleagues and may also serve to advocate for your client and persuade colleagues to adopt a particular view of the client's needs. Treatment plans, or self-management programs, explain to a patient how to do something (for example, how to perform a series of exercises or self-care procedures at home). Technical reports describe a procedure and explain how to execute it. Public health reports may include the planning or evaluation of a community health education intervention program. Each of these purposes of writing has a particular style or genre.

Table 4.1 Writing problems in order of importance and ways of addressing them

Writing problem	Proposed solution	Examples
1. Vague language	Make language clear and specific.	• Avoid sentences starting with 'This + (verb)', such as 'This had several consequences.' Always use a noun to explain what 'this' is referring to; for example, 'This decision had several consequences.'
2. Poor general vocabulary	Use words correctly and expand your vocabulary.	• Use a dictionary to clarify the meaning of a word when you are unsure of its exact meaning. If you have thought of a word but believe it is not the most appropriate one, use a thesaurus to find words with similar or related meanings. You can use the thesaurus on your computer. • Look at your references to see the words used in them.
3. Information not connected to point being made	Ensure that all information is relevant to the topic of the paragraph or section.	• Make sure every paragraph keeps to the topic announced or implied in its first sentence. • Use a new heading to signal a complete change of topic.
4. Wordiness (too many words)	Be concise; use short, clear sentences.	• An expression such as 'The problems which have been outlined in section 3 …' can be condensed to 'The problems outlined in section 3 …'. • An expression such as 'They studied the effect that dehydration had on …' can be condensed to 'They studied dehydration effects on …'. • The words in italics in the following expressions can usually be omitted without loss of meaning: 'It is *very* important to …'; 'Subjects detailed their *own* reactions to …'.
5. Important points not highlighted	Make sure important points are clear.	• List or state your key point(s), perhaps in an introductory sentence. • Write more about the points that are most important. • Write about the most important points first. • Explain why they are important.
6. Illogical reasoning	Be sure that your reasoning is clearly explained.	• After you have provided the necessary background information (e.g. information from other people's writings, information from observation of a patient, or information from your research), you should draw conclusions that are supported by that information. Explain why you think the conclusions are justified. • If you disagree with some information or interpretation, explain why with reference to the data provided.

Table 4.1 Writing problems in order of importance and ways of addressing them   (continued)

Writing problem	Proposed solution	Examples
7. Too much technical language	Use vocabulary that is generally understood; if you need to use technical language, define these terms.	• Take into account which words your intended audience should understand. Remember that much health science terminology is unfamiliar to lay people. If you have to use a technical word in a document for lay readers, explain what it means in simple words the first time you use it (e.g. 'Mr Smith has had a right cerebrovascular accident—that is, a stroke.') • Abbreviations that are familiar to you (e.g. CPR) may not be familiar to your readers. Always explain an abbreviation the first time you use it (e.g. 'CPR, or cardio-pulmonary resuscitation').
8. Poor overall organisation of writing	Organise your writing to help the reader understand the sequence of ideas.	• Make a plan of your writing (see Chapter 5). • Use headings as signposts to aid your readers. • Use different levels of headings to indicate when subtopics are nested within more major topics.
9. No clear overview	Include a clear overview.	• At the beginning of the document (essay, report, thesis, etc.), outline what is covered in that document. This gives readers an idea of what to expect, and helps them keep in mind an overview of the whole project.
10. Lacks continuity	Use strategies that maintain continuity of thought within and between paragraphs.	• Use linkages between sentences and paragraphs, such as 'The problems described above have several consequences, which can be divided into individual and community consequences. Among the individual consequences, … .'
11. Writing not adapted to audience	Adapt writing to suit the intended audience.	• When you come across new words in your lectures, practical work, or reading, it can be difficult to know if they are new just to you or if they would be unfamiliar to most non-specialists. Similarly, when people with English as a first language use a colloquial term, it can be difficult to know where that term can be used and for which audience. If this is a problem for you, ask lecturers and tutors for help. Ask your friends to explain the meaning of colloquial terms and their appropriate usage. In general, prefer simple, straightforward language. • See also point 7 above.
12. Poor grammar	Ensure grammar is correct.	• Work to improve your grammatical usage. Refer to style guidebooks. If you receive feedback on your writing, make a list of the rules that have been highlighted in this way, so you can refer to them when writing in the future.

Building basic writing skills

Students learning to write in English have some common problems, whether English is their first or second (or third!) language. Huckin and Olson (1991) outlined a variety of writing problems identified by senior professionals in science and industry. The most significant of these problems, and ways of addressing them, are shown in order of importance in Table 4.1.

Your education before university may not have emphasised English grammar, particularly if you are a student whose first language is not English. In Table 4.2 we provide some common rules of grammar. A frequent difficulty in English expression, especially for those whose first language is not English, is the use of *the English article* ('a/an', or 'the', or no article at all). For others, use of the numerous forms of *verb tense* is an unsolved mystery. If you can identify which aspects of English are specially difficult for you, staff at a learning support centre can suggest ways of getting help, or you can read a book on grammar and writing skills.

Table 4.2   Some basic rules of grammar

Rule	Example
A singular noun subject takes a singular verb in the present tense. That verb commonly has –s added to it.	Wilson (1998) *describes* the behaviour of institutionalised children.
A plural noun subject takes a plural verb in the present tense. That verb does not have –s added to it.	Jones and Potter (1997) *describe* the functions of diet.
A singular human noun is subsequently referred to using the words *he, him, his,* and *who* (for males) or *she, her, hers,* and *who* (for females).	Wilson (1998), *who* describes the behaviour of institutionalised children, gives *her* views on the causes …
A singular nonhuman noun is subsequently referred to using the words *it, its,* and *which*.	The diet, *which* is followed for four days, has as *its* main characteristic …
A plural noun is subsequently referred to using the words *they, them,* and *their*. Further, the referent used is *who* for human and *which* for nonhuman nouns.	Jones and Potter (1997), *who* describe the functions of diet, outline *their* program for …
The first time a noun is used, it is often prefaced by the article *a* (or *an* if it starts with a vowel). When mentioned again it is prefaced by the article *the*.	It is often effective to present your research in the form of *a* poster. *The* poster should be eye-catching and informative.
'a' refers to one or any (noun). 'the' refers to the specific or particular (noun).	Mr Smith has *an* eye disease … *The* disease may require treatment using …
As a general rule, keep the tense constant in a paragraph: use all past tense or all present tense as appropriate.	The patient *reported* that he had not eaten since last week. He *said* …

The effect of culture on writing

Culture affects writing in a variety of ways. Sentence structure and length, grammar, and vocabulary selection may all show the influence of cultural preferences in relation to formality, directness, and conceptual density of expression. As with face-to-face communication, levels of politeness used in writing also vary from culture to culture. Western Anglo professionals would be embarrassed by a referral letter that began *Dear Esteemed Colleague* or *Honoured Doctor*. However, such formal titles are appropriate in some cultures. The level of directness in writing also varies with the 'politeness demands' of cultures. Huckin and Olsen (1991) noted that Japanese writers prefer to slowly lay the groundwork for their main points throughout the letter or report, leaving the main points to the end, if indeed they are made at all. Readers are often left to draw their own conclusions rather than be 'told' or directed. According to Huckin and Olsen (p. 406), 'although a short, to-the-point letter may be very readable in the sense of being quickly understood, it may also be seen as somewhat curt and thus somewhat impolite by a Japanese'. However, Westerners tend to make main points and recommendations early in a report, or even at the start in the executive summary. You need to learn how to write appropriately for the situation (e.g. your university and country of enrolment).

The writing process: The 10 P's of academic writing

A common device in scholarly writing is to plan your writing around asking the following simple questions: Who ...? What ...? When ...? Where ...? Why ...? How ...? So what ...? These questions can be translated into various parameters (the 10 P's) of academic writing: people, purpose, preparation, principles, process, progression, position, product, proofing, presentation (see Table 4.3).

Table 4.3   The 10 P's of academic writing (© J. Higgs 2004)

	Meaning	**Guidelines**
People	Who is the author? Who is the audience?	• As author, consider your views and attitudes and how these might influence your writing. • Identify your target audience and how you should write for them: formal/informal language, expected knowledge, level of language, etc.
Purpose	Why am I writing? What is the goal of my paper or thesis?	• Use different styles/approaches to explain, persuade, and debate. • Identify your goals and match your content and style to them.
Preparation	How can I investigate this topic? How should I sort and store the information and data I collect? What are the findings of my research or topic investigation?	• Consider what fields of literature you need to investigate, what information and data you need to collect. • Spend time searching library catalogues to investigate your topic. • Set a time-frame that will help you get the task completed on time. • Develop a system for sorting, collating, and filing your data so that you can access the data easily when writing the various sections of the paper.

Table 4.3   The 10 P's of academic writing (© J. Higgs 2004)   (continued)

	Meaning	Guidelines
Principles	What are the rules of academic writing and referencing? What style/requirements are set by the school/discipline?	• Write with academic honesty. • Reference appropriately and avoid plagiarism. • Clearly indicate primary and secondary sources of ideas and quotes. • Identify the writing style and product required by your school or discipline. • Critique your work and that of authors you are referencing.
Process	How can I turn my ideas and information into a paper?	• Plan the content of the paper with such strategies as brainstorming and using a 'table of contents', flowcharts, and concept maps. • Write each planned section.
Progression	How can I structure the argument throughout the paper?	• Build the argument throughout the paper. • Create a structure or framework for the paper. • Build structure, flow, and connections into the paper at macro and micro levels.
Position	What is the point I am trying to make?	• Identify the position you wish to defend or the argument you wish to make and ensure that it is clearly expressed.
Product	What is the product of my writing: an essay? a journal article? a thesis? At the end of my work, how do I answer the 'So what?' question?	• Consider the preferred or required mode of presenting the argument or content. • What place do stories, examples, graphs, tables, models, pictures, etc., have in illustrating the argument? • What are the implications of your work for future research, education, and practice (if these are applicable)?
Proofing	What fine-tuning or checking is needed to finalise the paper?	• Before finishing your paper, essay, or thesis you should proofread it to check for clarity, sense, coherence, and technical correctness (e.g. accurate referencing, spelling, and grammar). • It helps to read your work aloud when proofing: incomplete sentences, lack of clarity, etc., become more evident this way.
Presentation	What are the presentation requirements and desired style of this work?	• Identify the expectations of this work in terms of presentation (e.g. word processing, length, and writing style). • Investigate what the typical thesis, essay, journal paper, etc., looks like for your field (e.g. headings, language, layout, and referencing style).

Essentially there are three parts to academic writing: the *big picture*, the *nitty gritty*, and the *process*. We will discuss each of these in detail.

The big picture

This refers to the fundamental argument or explanation you are presenting. For this task you need to consider the *people*, *purpose*, *progression*, *position*, and *product* items from Table 4.3. In crafting your argument, remember to structure your work. Firstly, this involves planning an overall structure. It may take the form of a logical sequence of headings or questions, or a standard research-report sequence including Introduction, Background Literature, Research Methods, Results and Conclusion. Secondly, within the argument you need to think about how you will create the flow of the argument or build your case. This entails:

- creating signposts by, for example, starting with your endpoint ('In this essay I argue that …') and then going on to make this argument
- using each paragraph to present a main idea and each section to make the next major point in your case
- linking the ideas, through a logical sequence or through linking phrases, such as 'Having presented the background to this topic, my next task is to …' and 'Based on these results …').

The nitty gritty

This refers to the technical aspects of writing, the details, and the presentation of your work (see *principles*, *proofing* and *presentation* in Table 4.3). With all the tools available today (e.g. word processing software, spell-checkers, online computer searches, style guides, and reference manuals) there is no reason why your work should not be well researched, well checked (with accurate referencing, spelling, grammar, and punctuation) and well presented. These aspects of your work are largely invisible if you do them well; they add a polish to your work. But if poorly done they are glaringly obvious and detract from your argument. Even the strongest case or the most interesting research can be tarnished by poor presentation or spelling, and your grade or the impact of your work could suffer. You may need to learn these skills or improve your basic writing skills. Most universities have student learning centres where you can seek such aid. Learning these skills is an essential part of your tertiary education. Table 4.4 provides some valuable technical guidelines for academic writing.

HANDY HINT ☞ **4.2 Resources for grammar and style**

Publication Manual of the American Psychological Association 2001, 5th edn, American Psychological Association, Washington, DC. Although this manual is designed primarily for writers of journal articles and theses, it has useful sections on writing style, grammar, and reducing bias in language. These sections deal with important matters that are subject to error in health and social sciences writing in general.

Zwier, L. J., 2002, *Building Academic Vocabulary*, The University of Michigan Press, Ann Arbor, Michigan. Addressing academic writing in particular, this book provides many synonyms for words commonly used in essays, assignments, theses, etc. Differences between similar terms are clearly explained, to help demonstrate the most appropriate usages.

Style Manual for Authors, Editors and Printers 2002, 6th edn, rev. by Snooks & Co., John Wiley & Sons Australia.

Tyler, S., Kossen, C., & Ryan, C., 2002, *Communication: A Foundation Course*, 2nd edn, Prentice Hall Australia, Sydney.

The process

See Table 4.3 for the *preparation* and *process* items. Table 4.4 provides some strategies to help you write well. Also refer to the other chapters in this book that focus on specific aspects of writing and preparation.

Conclusion

At the end of your writing, it is time to reflect on the process of your writing and its product. Consider, for example, the following questions:

- Have you said what you wanted to say? Have you made your message clear?
- Did you complete your task (e.g. to critique, explain, debate, discuss, or report)?
- What have you learned about your writing? What skills might you need to develop?
- What are the strengths and weaknesses of your writing?

Turner (2002) listed the criteria to use in assessing the quality of essays: structure, clarity of thought, evidence of reading, coherence of argument, and presentation quality. Have you addressed all of these criteria?

References

Huckin, T. N. & Olsen, L. A. 1991, *Technical Writing and Professional Communication for Nonnative Speakers of English* (international edn), McGraw Hill, New York.

Turner, J. 2002, *How to Study: A Short Introduction*, Sage Publications, London.

Further reading

Arnold, J., Poston, C. & Witek, K. 1999, *Research Writing in the Information Age*, Allyn and Bacon, Boston, Massachusetts.

Bate, D. & Sharpe, P. 1996, *Student Writer's Handbook for University Students*, Harcourt Brace, Sydney.

Bazerman, C. & Weiner, H. S. 1998, *Writing Skills Handbook*, 4th edn, Houghton Mifflin, Boston.

Burnard, P. 1997, *Effective Communication Skills for Health Professionals*, 2nd edn, Stanley Thornes, Cheltenham, UK.

Cormack, D. F. S. 1994, *Writing for Health Care Professionals*, Blackwell Scientific, Oxford.

Creme, P. & Lea, M. R. 1997, *Writing at University: A Guide for Students*, Open University Press, Buckingham.

Fergusson, R. (ed.) 1986, *The Penguin A–Z Thesaurus*, Penguin Books, London.

Holliday, A. 2002, *Doing and Writing Qualitative Research*, Sage Publications, London.

Li, X. & Crane, N. 1993, *Electronic Style: A Guide to Citing Electronic Information*, Meckler, Westport.

Lindsay, D. 1995, *A Guide to Scientific Writing*, 2nd edn, Longman, Melbourne.

Ludowyk, F. & Moore, B. 1999, *The Australian Oxford Paperback Dictionary*, 3rd edn, Oxford University Press, Melbourne.

Macquarie Dictionary <http://www.macquariedictionary.com.au/> accessed 17 July 2003.

Oxford English Dictionary <http://www.oed.com/> accessed 17 July 2003.

Peat, J., Elliott, E., Baur, L. & Keenan, V. 2002, *Scientific Writing: Easy When You Know How*, BMJ Books, Sydney.

Ritter, R. M. 2003, *The Oxford Style Manual: The Essential Handbook for All Writers, Editors, and Publishers*, Oxford University Press, Oxford.

Roget's Thesaurus <http://thesaurus.reference.com/Roget-Alpha-Index.html> accessed 17 July 2003.

Style Manual for Authors, Editors and Printers 2002, 6th edn, rev. by Snooks & Co., John Wiley & Sons Australia.

Wallace, A., Schirato, T. & Bright, P. 1999, *Beginning University: Thinking, Researching and Writing for Success*, Allen & Unwin, St Leonards, NSW.

Table 4.4 Technical aspects of writing

Task/item	Guidelines
Writing style, punctuation, and grammar	• Writing style is a combination of general expectations of academic writing (these are essential) and local instructions (e.g. university style requirements and specific-essay instructions).
	• See the section earlier in this chapter on 'Characteristics of academic writing'. In particular, concentrate on clarity of expression and message, and avoid long sentences and distracting layout and terminology.
	• Grammar and punctuation should be accurate: not only is this required for academic writing, it is also an indication of the literacy and education of the writer.
Spelling	• Use the Australian rather than American spelling of words like 'honour', 'practise' (the verb), 'equalled', and 'organise' (except, of course, when writing for American journals). However, when quoting, retain the original spelling.
	• Set your software spell-checker to Australian or British spelling.
	• Choose or follow local instructions about spelling options, but be consistent (except for spelling within quotes) (for example, 'program' or 'programme', 'aging' or' ageing', '–ise' or '–ize').
Font	• Use a font that is easy to read and not distracting, such as Times New Roman (TNR) or Arial. A font with serifs (such as TNR) is easier to read in block text, like paragraphs, than a font without serifs (such as Arial). Avoid distracting the reader with fancy fonts. Use 12 point (= Arial 10), or 11 if there is a need to save space.
	• Use italics for emphasis.
	• Use quotation marks or italics when you are citing new or jargon terms for the first time. Add a footnote or endnote with a definition, or explain the term in the text.
	• Don't use underlining; italicise if there is a need for emphasis.
	• Use bold for headings only, not for emphasis.
Layout and printing (general)	• The aesthetics of your presentation/layout is a matter of taste. Make sure you follow any set requirements for your work: check your university's guide for presentation of assignments. Beyond that, make the text readable, the graphics clear, and the overall appearance scholarly. Sometimes there is a place for more creative layout (e.g. posters with graphics).
	• The layout of your writing (e.g. heading levels and paragraph breaks) has 'hidden meanings': the reader will assume that each paragraph is a new point, each same-level heading begins a section of equal importance, and so on. Recognise and use this factor.
	• Avoid wasteful and distracting white space; avoid one-sentence or very small paragraphs (they stop the flow of the argument).

Table 4.4 Technical aspects of writing   (continued)

Task/item	Guidelines
Layout and printing (general) (continued)	• Justification refers to the left- and right-side alignment of your text. Left-sided justification is standard in the main text and should be used in most tables. Double (right and left) justification can be used for standard block text. In tables, right-justify or decimal-justify numbers, and include a consistent number of decimal places or use decimal tabs. • 'Portrait' page layout is most common and expected. Sometimes, as with a wide table (such as this one), horizontal or 'landscape' page layout is preferable. • Check the spacing requirements for your paper. You may need to use double spacing or wide margins (for thesis binding, etc.). • Different printers space text differently. A page of text from one printer may expand to a page and 3 lines on another. Check the layout on the monitor before your final print, especially if you are using manual page breaks. • When possible, use laser printing, particularly for theses. Otherwise use clear (not faint or hard-to-read) print and printers.
Headings	• You may use the heading system built into your software (see the section on style sheets in Chapter 16). • Here is an example of a system of headings: > Chapter/essay title—centred, capitals, bold, font size 16, 2 paragraph spaces after > Major text headings—left-justified, bold, capitals, 2 paragraph spaces before, 1 after > Second-level text headings—left-justified, bold, sentence case, 1 paragraph space before, 0 after > Third-level text headings—left-justified, italics, not bold, sentence case, 1 paragraph space before, 0 after • Avoid complex section numbering, such as 3.2.2.3. It is hard to follow.
Headers, footers, page numbers, and tabs	• Headers and footers may be used if acceptable, but are generally used only in drafts, to keep track of the version/date of updating. • Use page numbers. • Use tabs rather than the space bar to ensure correct alignment of text.
Footnotes and endnotes	• Footnotes (bottom of page) or endnotes (end of document) may be used to add information (e.g. definitions) that is not necessary in the text or slows down the flow of the argument. • Check if such notes are acceptable, but do not use too many; they make the document hard to read. • Many software programs allow you to insert these notes systematically, with sequenced numbers that adjust automatically if new notes are added.

Table 4.4 Technical aspects of writing (continued)

Task/item	Guidelines
Tables and figures	• See Chapter 17.
Lists	• In general, avoid using lists in essays, because they do not create a sense of flow or build up the argument, and often the message is obscured in the more cryptic and staccato style created by lists, bullet points, etc. Sometimes lists may usefully be placed in tables for reference, rather than as the main part of the text/argument. • For an indented series of points, use numbers—(1), (2), etc.—only if the sequence is important. If the sequence is not significant use bullets. Use balance in the grammatical presentation of your points. For example, if the first point starts with a verb ending with '–ing', all the other points in that series should start the same way. • Delineation of a series of points within a sentence can be clarified for the reader by use of (a), (b), (c), etc. Use a comma between each point unless the points already have commas within them, in which case you should use semicolons.
Numerals and dates	• Write out in words all numbers less than 10, and numbers starting a sentence. However, use figures for numbers relating to any unit of measurement (e.g. 6 months). • Use a consistent date format, such as day–month–year (e.g. 15 August 1993). • Decades are written without an apostrophe (e.g. 1980s, not 1980's).
Use of the first person ('I', 'me', 'we', etc.)	• This usage is becoming more accepted in academic writing in appropriate instances, such as when the writer needs to acknowledge the part that his or her involvement played in the study's outcome. At other times the convention is to use the passive voice, as in 'Several factors were taken into consideration in designing the layout of the room.' But excessive usage of the passive voice can sound both detached and convoluted. • Check if there are any local rules that apply to your institution regarding use of the first person. Some institutions stipulate writing in the third person.
Singular/plural	• Singular subjects are accompanied by singular verbs; plural subjects take plural verbs. • Avoid using singular nouns like 'the nurse' and then having to use 'his/her'. It is preferable to say 'nurses … their …'.
Tense	• Use the past tense to report what researchers/authors found, studied, reported, claimed, considered, etc. • When writing up your research methods, change the future tense ('I will …'/'This research will investigate …') of your research proposal to the past tense ('I did …'/'This research investigated …')

Table 4.4 Technical aspects of writing (continued)

Task/item	Guidelines
Inanimate/animate subjects	• There are some verbs that do not fit with inanimate subjects. Only animate subjects (researchers, authors, theorists, etc.) can discuss, contend, claim, assert, consider, argue, or aim to. Inanimate subjects (studies, research, findings, chapters, theses, etc.) can demonstrate, present, provide, and so on.
Abbreviations and jargon	• Use a full stop after abbreviations that do not end with the same letter as the word (e.g. 'Prof.' and 'Fig.'). • Don't use a full stop after abbreviations that end with the same letter as the word (e.g. 'Dr' and 'Figs'). • Note the use of full stops in the following abbreviations: 'etc.', 'i.e.', 'e.g.', 'et al.' • Explain technical terms and abbreviations the first time they are used. This can be in the text or in a footnote (if acceptable). In longer works, like theses, a glossary of technical terms may be worth including.
Referencing and quotes	• See Chapter 7.

05 | LEARNING TO WRITE ESSAYS AND ASSIGNMENTS

Iain Hay and Lindy McAllister

KEY TOPICS

→ How to analyse an essay topic

→ How to structure an essay

→ How to support your case

→ How to write well

Introduction

Writing is one of the most powerful means we have of communicating. It is also a thought-provoking, generative process that offers us the opportunity to present our work to others and seek feedback on our ideas. A good essay must clearly set out *what you think and what you have learned about a specific topic* (Hay et al. 2002, p. 67). The pages that follow are intended to help you achieve this end. The chapter provides advice on analysing your essay topic, structuring your essay, supporting your case, and writing well.

Analysing the topic

A good essay *answers the question assigned* and deals in detail with the specific issues the topic raises. These matters are absolutely critical to essay-writing success. There are several steps you can take to ensure that you are on the right track.

First, read the essay topic through carefully, underlining or highlighting key words within it, as shown in the example below:

Write an essay that <u>discusses</u> the <u>effects</u> of <u>recent private health-insurance rebates</u> for the <u>public health-care sector</u> in <u>Australia</u>.

Second, dissect each of the key words and their relationships with others in the essay statement. Essay assignments commonly ask you to examine, discuss, explore, explain, compare, contrast, analyse, critique, etc. Look up these words in a good dictionary to ensure you know what they mean. The word 'discuss' here implies that you need to 'examine the subject matter critically'. Think about the word 'effects' in this essay assignment. What kinds of effect? The topic makes it clear that the paper should deal with effects on the public health-care sector. But does this mean, for example, effects on the ways in which health-care services are delivered in remote areas? on the type and frequency of services available? on the length and duration of public health-care waiting lists? on public-sector funding? on working conditions for medical staff? In this assignment, the specific area is unclear. You have at least two options in such a case:

- You could speak to your lecturer or tutor and ask if there are any specific issues you should be focusing on. It might help to be prepared to suggest to your teacher some of the areas you would like to cover if such scope exists.
- You could make it clear in your essay that while a wide range of effects could be considered, you are choosing to focus on specific ones because of the length constraints of the essay. You must justify that selection. Make it clear why, for instance, you are discussing waiting lists and not relative funding flows to the public and private sectors under the new rebates structure.

Finally, it is evident from the topic that the paper must deal with Australia as a whole and not some small part of it (e.g. NSW or Victoria). While you can use local examples and case studies to illustrate particular points, you must keep the national context as the focus.

The third step in preparing to write a good essay is learning (more) about your topic. The recommended texts and reading lists for your subject are a good start, but on most occasions you will need to read more widely. This will require judicious literature searching and careful reference management. These matters are dealt with fully in Chapters 6 and 7. As you read, you should make useful notes (noting when quotes are taken) and record the source of all the information and data you collect. Refer to Chapter 3 about academic honesty and avoiding plagiarism.

5.1   Exploring an essay topic

When investigating your topic area, focus your reading on the topic (avoid wasting time reading too widely) and read critically. Ask yourself, 'Is this material credible? Is this relevant to my topic or the argument I am trying to make?'

HANDY HINT

Structuring your essay

There are many levels at which you can consider the structure of an essay. At the global level, all good essays typically comprise three main parts: introduction, body, and conclusion. A good essay has a logical order of content that supports the argument or answer the essay is presenting.

Introduction

In the introduction you should do at least four things. First, state your topic, purpose, and 'case'. Let the reader know clearly what the essay is about. However, whatever you do, *do not* simply restate the essay question as the statement of intent. For instance, if the assigned essay question is 'Write an essay that discusses the effects of recent private health insurance rebates for the public health-care sector in Australia', do not start with a statement like 'This essay discusses the effects of recent private health insurance rebates for the public health-care sector in Australia.' You might find greater success with something that grabs the reader's attention, in the form, perhaps, of an amazing statistic, an anecdote, or a controversial statement that focuses on some key element of your essay. For example, your paper might begin as follows: 'Since the Federal Government introduced its private health insurance rebate public health system, reform of the system has been blocked and the system now faces ruin without major cash inputs.' This highlights the second function of a good introduction: it captures the reader's attention. Third, the introduction should explain the significance of the topic. Why is this matter important? Who cares? What is affected by this? Answers to these questions will give you a strong lead into identifying the significance of your work. Finally, a good introduction will usually provide a 'map' of the discussion to follow. Give your reader some idea of the intellectual journey you have planned for them.

Essay body

The body of the essay is the place where you set out the reasons and evidence for the case or views you introduced earlier. You must substantiate each of your claims. If we return to the claim made earlier in our example essay that the Australian public health system 'now faces ruin without major cash inputs', you will have to provide statistical evidence, quotes from experts, or other evidence to support this claim. You should also consider using figures, tables, plates, and maps as proof of your case. Without good evidence, your assertions will never be anything more than that.

Conclusion

The third and final part of an essay is the conclusion. Here you should distil the essence of your answer to the question posed. The conclusion must be based on evidence set out within the body of the paper. It is not a place for new material or the 'surprise witness'. The conclusion needs also to be related logically to the introduction. Make sure the conclusion matches the intent indicated in the introduction.

Developing your structure

A good essay has a coherent conceptual structure within which examples, evidence, and argument are placed. You might imagine the structure as a skeleton and the evidence as the flesh. Both are needed, and in the right combination, to complete the essay. There are two particularly useful techniques for developing an essay's internal structure: the essay plan and the sketch diagram.

Essay plan

To prepare an essay plan, you need to have a clear idea of the general argument you wish to make in your essay before you start writing it. With this general argument in mind, make a list of the major headings you might use to describe material in different parts of the essay.

Then look at their order. Rearrange them if necessary. Then, under each heading, add a series of subheadings and, under those, ideas for references, data, and the like. Work like this until you have a detailed plan of the essay framework and of the kind of points you need to make in each section and the reference materials you need to support your claims. Most word processing packages include options (e.g. outline view) that will help you develop an essay plan.

Sketch diagram

If you have a less clear idea about the direction you wish to take in your essay, you could start your planning by drawing a sketch diagram or flowchart. Jot down on a sheet of paper all of the key words and ideas you can think of that relate to the essay topic. Eliminate any duplication. Diagram the content, drawing connections between elements. Keep rearranging your diagram until you feel you have generated an essay outline. You can then use this as the foundation for an essay plan.

Free writing

If neither of these strategies works there is another, sometimes more time-consuming and frustrating approach you can adopt: free writing. Simply start writing something related to the topic. The key idea here is to get words on paper or screen. Once there, the words can be edited, rearranged, and otherwise massaged into the form of an essay. This approach should normally be one of last resort. It is usually easier and more productive to plan an essay and then write than it is to write and then plan! (It is also important to note that it is much easier to plan, map, or free-write after you have done preliminary reading on the topic you are trying to write about!)

Using headings for clarity and structure

Your completed essay may include headings throughout to help readers follow the flow of the argument and to allow them to return to any specific section quickly. As the discussion of essay planning above suggests, headings are also useful organisational tools. For instance, once you have completed a draft of your paper, write out on a separate sheet of paper all the headings you plan to use. Separated from the content of the essay, does the order of headings make sense, following a logical sequence that contributes to a good essay answer? If not, think about rearranging the headings or adding or deleting headings (and therefore sections in your essay). Once you are satisfied with the order of the headings, revisit the text of your essay, rearranging it to match the framework you have devised. You may find that your summary of headings provides a helpful framework for your essay's introduction.

It is sometimes necessary to use a hierarchy of headings in an essay. Generally, three levels is sufficient but in rare cases up to five may be needed. The suggestions for formatting headings in Handy Hint 5.2 may be useful (see page 46).

Supporting your case thoroughly

Claims, contentions, arguments, and allegations in an essay all require the support of high-quality evidence or argument. This is material such as data, quotations, examples, and case studies that substantiate the case or position you are trying to put forward in your essay. Do not make assertions or generalisations (e.g. 'Women who have children young have a lower risk than older first-time mothers of getting breast cancer') without including facts to back them up.

BOLD CAPITALS

MEDIUM CAPITALS

MEDIUM ITALIC CAPITALS

CAPITALS AND SMALL CAPITALS

or

BOLD CAPITALS

Bold lower case

Bold italic lower case

Italic lower case

Italic lower case. With text running on...

or

BOLD CAPITALS

Bold Upper and Lower Case

Bold italic lower case

Italic lower case

Reference material

A good essay will demonstrate that you have referred to and considered work written by others in related fields. Many first and second year students in particular express concern that they do not know enough about a topic to be able to write an essay about it and so feel condemned to do little more than quote the work of others. It is worth bearing in mind that no project springs from a vacuum. We all rely to some extent on the work of others who have gone before. To think otherwise is to deny the value of any sense of scientific 'progress' (i.e. incremental development of knowledge). What this means, in part, is that all of the work we do, either as new students or as senior scholars in a field, requires us to use and *interpret* the available literature to answer a specific question. So, use the references that are available to help you think critically about the writing task you have been assigned. Do not parrot the ideas you find. A good essay assignment will probably not allow you to do this anyway; instead, it might require you to think of ways in which the work of other people 'informs' your study. Let us say, for example, that you are writing an essay on the reasons behind community protests about the opening of a new mental health facility in Remuera, a well-to-do inner-city suburb of Auckland. You are unlikely to find much in the way of literature on 'mental health facilities in Remuera'. However, there will certainly be reference material on the location of similar facilities elsewhere, on community protests, and so on. You need to look for that sort of material and make appropriate connections between it and your work.

Students commonly ask, 'How many references do I need?' There is no right answer to this question. Except in the rare cases where there is no extant body of literature, or you have been asked to write an unsubstantiated 'opinion piece', your examiner will expect to see some references cited. If you have not received guidelines on the number of references to use, decide this by considering whether there are many or few good references on this topic in the literature and how long the essay should be. In general, use fewer references for short essays. Like the rest of the evidence you employ, your references should be *relevant, reputable, accurate, up-to-date, and sufficient to support your case*. Such sources include, for example, scholarly books and refereed journals (such as *Advances in Speech Language Pathology*, *Australian Journal of Physiotherapy*, *Research in Developmental Disabilities*, *The Lancet*, and *The Medical Journal of Australia*). A refereed journal is one in which the contents have been scrutinised carefully by referees who are experts in the field, before being accepted for publication. In general, poor-quality or inaccurate papers are rejected by the referees and are not published. Most refereed journals include in their 'instructions to authors' (often found on the inside covers) a statement to the effect that manuscripts are sent to referees for comment. Websites may also be useful, particularly those produced by professional bodies (e.g. the sites of the American Speech-Language and Hearing Association and the Australian Medical Association). However, when you are considering using Web material to support your essay, be very sceptical of sources until you have checked the website out. There are several matters you might wish to consider when evaluating the value of a website for your work (Curtin University School of Public Health 2001):

- *Scope*. Does the site offer the information you really need? For example, is it about the right country? Does it relate directly to your essay topic or is it of marginal relevance?
- *Purpose and presentation*. What is the reason for the site's existence? Is the information likely to be biased? Is the site well organised and is the material presented clearly?
- *Authority*. Who are the authors and what are their claims to credibility?
- *Currency and content*. When was the site produced? Are sources of information acknowledged?

If you have any doubts about the credibility of the site and the information within it, you would be best to ignore it. At the very least you should critique all of your sources and referenced material.

5.3   Consider the reliability of Web information

When you are searching the Web for reference material, remember that anyone with access to a networked computer can publish on the Web and there is no requirement whatsoever that anything disseminated there be true, or that it be peer-reviewed like material in refereed journals. Be particularly wary of websites and webpages that have no clearly identified institutional or individual author.

HANDY HINT

When you write an essay it is important that you acknowledge the thoughts and efforts of others upon whose work you have built your own project. You can achieve this by fully and correctly citing the source details of quotations, evidence, and ideas, using an accepted form of referencing or professional acknowledgment. To fail to do so will probably be interpreted as plagiarism, a form of intellectual theft. A good essay also includes a complete and correctly presented list of references. Be sure that all the references you cite in your essay are acknowledged fully in footnotes or the reference list and that you properly use an accepted form of referencing. Some universities have an 'in-house' referencing system, and in some professional courses students are advised to follow the style guide used by journals in the discipline. For example, because speech pathology journals commonly use the Publication Manual of the American Psychological Association (2001), speech pathology students in some universities are encouraged to follow that guide. If there is any aspect of referencing conventions that you do not understand, seek clarification from your lecturer.

Illustrative material

Plates, figures, tables, and maps are often overlooked as useful illustrative or evidentiary devices in essays. Illustrations can be derived from other sources or you can create your own; for example, for an essay on the positive and negative consequences of acupuncture as a treatment for premenstrual pain, you might prepare a summary table set out in two columns, one for 'pros' and the other for 'cons'. Make sure that your illustrations support, not 'talk for', the text. Remember that your key argument should be in the text.

HANDY HINT ☞ **5.4   Finding images on the Internet**

Internet search engines can be a useful source of photographs and other images for your essays. For instance, Google provides a very simple image-search tool that uses exactly the same key-word functions as its normal text-based searches. Subject to copyright laws and other relevant institutional regulations, images may be copied and pasted into your own document. You must, of course, acknowledge the source of the images in your work. This image-search feature can be useful if you need pictures that you could not be expected to obtain otherwise (e.g. a photograph of a health-care clinic in Bolivia).

Tables, figures, and the like can often make a point much better than you can make it in words; after all, 'a picture is worth a thousand words'. However, when you do use illustrative material, be sure it is accurate and germane to the case you are making. Do not fill your paper with pretty pictures and tables of marginal relevance. The different kinds of illustrations and the labels you should give them in papers are shown in Table 5.1.

Table 5.1 Types of illustrative material and their labels

Type of material	Label
Graphs, diagrams, and maps	Figure
Tables	Table
Photographs	Figure (sometimes labelled Plate)

You should also ensure that you refer within the text of your essay to every illustration (for example, with a statement like 'see Table 3') and that each illustration is self-contained. This means that someone can look at the table or figure and know what it is about without having to read the text of your essay to work it out. Unless your lecturer advises you otherwise, place illustrative material as close as possible to the section where you first refer to it. It should not be located at the end of your essay or in a set of appendices, for it needs to be close to the argument or point it is intended to support. You will find more detailed advice on preparing graphics and tables in Chapter 17.

Writing well

Good written expression is critical to essay success. You can become a better writer by (a) practising writing, (b) following some simple principles, and (c) listening to constructive criticism. Writing a good, well-expressed essay also takes time. Do not be fooled into thinking that your first essay draft is the final copy. It is vital that you allow yourself the opportunity both to do ample research and to write and rewrite drafts of your paper. A good essay is rarely written on the first attempt.

Short sentences

One of the simplest ways to ensure that your essay is written fluently is to keep the sentences short. Have a look at essays you have written in the past and any you are currently working on. How long are the sentences? If you find that you make a habit of creating sentences longer than 25 words you are probably running the risk of creating grammatical minefields that are difficult and frustrating to read. To avoid such problems, try keeping sentences on the first draft of your essay to about 10–20 words. Chop long sentences up. Express ideas simply. Express them succinctly. You will probably find that short sentences are not only easier to manage as you write but that they have greater impact too.

Effective paragraphing

Another key to good essay writing is effective paragraphing. A paragraph is typically a self-contained expression of a single main idea. It generally consists of three parts. The first is a *topic sentence*. This introduces or states the main idea. For instance, 'Like many countries in the developed world, Australia has an aging population.' The second part is the *supporting sentence or sentences*. These provide evidence to support the topic sentence. For example, 'In 1961, only 8.5% of the population was over 65 years of age, whereas by 2031 it is anticipated that figure will have increased to 22%.' The third and final part of a paragraph is known as the *clincher*. Following through with our example, we might conclude the paragraph with a statement like this: 'Australia's changing demographic profile has important implications for health-service planning and delivery.' Although it is true that not all paragraphs contain these three components, you will probably find that an awareness of this structure is highly valuable as you develop your essay-writing abilities.

One difficulty many people face when writing an essay is trying to link one paragraph to another. Without good links an essay can sometimes read rather like a sequence of related ideas rather than as a coherent, single work. Some useful phrases to help bind one paragraph to another include the following:

Another matter to consider is …	*Elsewhere …*
On the other hand …	*Other common …*
A similar explanation …	*A significant consequence is …*
From a different perspective…	*A number of issues can be identified …*

Grammar and punctuation

Difficulties with grammar and punctuation often trip up otherwise good students (see Chapter 4). There are two main steps you can take to improve both the fluency and grammatical accuracy of your papers.

First, if you are confused about matters such as the correct location of an apostrophe or the right time to use a colon as opposed to a semi-colon, *don't guess*. Find out and learn!

There are many good books on these subjects. And even if you think you have highly developed grammatical abilities, you might still find it worth consulting texts such as Peters' (1995) *The Cambridge Australian English Style Guide* or Greenbaum's (1996) *The Oxford English Grammar* for advice.

Second, once you have written a paper and believe it is complete, put it aside for a few days. When you come back to it you will probably be able to read it more critically than when the words were typed fresh on the screen. All of a sudden you will see odd phrasings, flaws in your argument, and typographical errors that simply were not there before! It can sometimes be helpful to have a good friend, one whose skills as a writer in your field you value, read through your essay, marking it as they go. You may be able to reciprocate, critically evaluating and commenting on their work. Another valuable idea is to read the paper aloud to yourself. This will help you identify clumsy constructions, repetition, and other problems. Alternatively, you could ask a friend to read the paper out aloud to you. This has two benefits. You will hear quickly where they have a problem following the structure by their audible slip-ups and mistakes as they try to articulate as best they can the text before them. It will also allow you to hear in someone else's voice the ideas you set down on paper, and to listen for problems (e.g. lack of clarity or coherence) that you need to address.

Spelling

With the advent of powerful spell-checkers in word processing programs, few excuses for spelling errors remain. However, you should always check the work of your computer! There are occasions when you will have to outsmart the machinery and provide it with guidance with words like bow and bough; two, too, and to; and affect and effect. Remember to attach the appropriate dictionary (e.g. Australian) to your file and set it as the default language on your computer for spell-checking.

HANDY HINT ☞   **5.5   Keep the original spelling in quotes**

When you are using your word processing spell-checking feature, be careful not to change the original spelling in quotes or references (e.g. from American to Australian English). That would be an error. If there is a spelling error in a quote, indicate this by '[sic]' after the misspelled word. Don't change the spelling.

You should also pay particular attention to technical terms. If you cannot correctly spell or use words that belong to your vocation, you cast into doubt your abilities in other professional domains. To assist you here, you could buy a good dictionary of medical terms or consult a reliable website of professional terminology. You may also need to define professional jargon terms, unless you can expect them to be readily understood by your reader(s).

Presentation and word limits

Take care with the presentation of your essays. An essay that is nicely typed and formatted in accordance with your lecturer's requirements will make a better first impression than one that is sloppily handwritten, dog-eared, and coffee-stained.

Most essays have a word limit. Stick to it. Some markers monitor word limits closely, arguing that students who exceed the specified word limit may have an unfair advantage over those who keep to it. Also, in a large class a hundred extra words on each essay quickly adds up to a lot of extra reading and marking. And that can make for a frustrated and unhappy marker! Make each word count. And if you find that you do not have enough words to meet the 'limit', you can either stop writing, having said all you need to, or (and this probably more advisable) you can to do some more research.

Conclusion

Writing essays and assignments is a skill that can be learned and refined with practice. Writing good essays and assignments takes time: time to analyse what is required, to plan out the writing task, and to structure it effectively. Time is also required to find references and other material to support your argument. Effective writing is also about paying attention to the details of spelling, punctuation, and grammar. Finally, you need to allow time for drafting (and redrafting) and for proofreading, so that your ideas and manner of expressing them can be fine-tuned. With good time management and regular practice you can learn to write essays and assignments that will be a pleasure to read and mark, and that demonstrate the depth and scope of your learning.

References

American Psychological Association 2001, *Publication Manual of the American Psychological Association*, 5th edn, American Psychological Association, Washington, DC.

Curtin University School of Public Health 2001, 'Online tutorial: Effectively searching and evaluating health information on the World Wide Web' <http://www.curtin.edu.au/curtin/dept/health/> accesssed 8 March 2004.

Greenbaum, S. 1996, *The Oxford English Grammar*, Oxford University Press, Oxford.

Hay, I., Bochner, D. & Dungey, C. 2002, *Making the Grade: A Guide to Successful Communication and Study*, Oxford University Press, Melbourne.

Peters, P. 1995, *The Cambridge Australian English Style Guide*, Cambridge University Press, Melbourne.

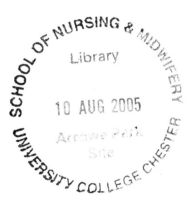

06 SEARCHING THE LITERATURE AND MANAGING THE COLLECTED DATA

Ann Sefton and Annette Street

KEY TOPICS

→ Determining the depth and range of searching required

→ Finding out what is already known about the topic

→ Locating relevant knowledge 'out there' electronically

→ Summarising and storing information from searches

Introduction

For at least two reasons, it is important to develop excellent literature-searching skills. First, a strong evidence base is essential for the health and social sciences. Second, skills in searching for, locating, and evaluating the relevance of information are important for learning. Teachers often provide reading lists of references to articles, books, chapters, and information on the Internet, which will help you to gain a deeper understanding.

6.1   Effective literature searching

HANDY HINT

- Use the resources supplied by the course convenor.
- Track down up-to-date references.
- Follow up citations and references from key articles.
- Distinguish between primary sources and secondary sources.
- Identify the amount and depth of discussion required in each assignment.
- Review the literature, don't retell it.
- Keep records of your searches.
- Be systematic in your storage of articles.
- Develop rigour in the skills of citation and referencing.

Most textbooks also list references at the end of each chapter or section to provide alternative explanations or more detail. You will find it helpful to consult these additional sources to understand difficult concepts or to explore interesting ideas further. It is also important to remember that there is a time lag between the generation of knowledge and its publication in textbooks. You may need to search for more recent references that have been published since the book was written. Reading beyond the set text can help you understand essential material so that you can later express your ideas and demonstrate your understanding confidently in class, or in oral or written presentations and examinations. As you progress through your program, you will increasingly be expected to draw conclusions from your reading, and to explain and defend them on the basis of the evidence you have collected.

When you have to complete an essay, talk, thesis, assignment, report, or project, you will need to locate and read relevant material. In particular, students who undertake honours or extension work will find that locating, reading, and interpreting the literature represents a major component of their study and assessment. Leave yourself enough time to do the necessary reading and thinking.

As you progress academically you are expected to become more independent in finding your own sources of information and to be more critical in interpreting them. You may also become more curious to follow up ideas that you find intriguing or difficult. It can become an absorbing task of scholarship to track the development of important ideas in the health and social sciences by following up references, seeing how subsequent authors contribute to a deeper understanding of particular issues. Occasionally you may even uncover examples of faulty logic or misinterpretation!

Locating information
Libraries

Even before coming to university, you will be familiar with searching for books in libraries. A large academic library, however, is much more complex than a typical local library or school library. Resources for different disciplines may well be stored in different buildings, even on separate campuses. You need to know how to find the right library, and the appropriate section within it. Library information sessions will be beneficial early in your program, even if you have been using smaller libraries for years.

Most books are indexed according to a standard bibliographic convention. The widely used Dewey system originally assigned a number between 1 and 1,000 to each topic or area, so that books and journals on similar topics are stored together. For example, books on dentistry usually have a Dewey number of 617, with the different sub-specialties distinguished by decimal places: orthodontics and paediatric dentistry are at 617.64; dental radiology is at 617.6623. Books relating to oral surgery may be found at 617.661, although books on certain aspects of that subject may be at 616.99431 (cancer of the mouth: 616.994 for cancer, 31 for mouth) with other books on medical pathology. Be aware that the numbers are updated over time, so you may need to consult the most recent cataloguing system to find the relevant book. The system is complex because of the constant proliferation of new subject areas and the difficulty of classifying items that cross subject boundaries. You may find that some libraries use their own systems for classifying and locating books and journals in special areas, so it is important to learn the particular features of the libraries you will be most likely to use. It is also crucial to become familiar with computer-based catalogues and databases, which can make your searches more efficient and save unnecessary journeys. They are usually very user-friendly.

HANDY HINT ☞ 6.2   Library Pathfinder Questions 1: How to locate *known* references

- What type of information carrier (e.g. whole book or periodical) am I looking for?
- What accurate information do I have about this reference?
- Which parts of the reference are the most useful to search for?
- Does this catalogue or database provide *Help* tools?
- Do I understand the basic search features in this catalogue or database?
- Have I selected the best search function in this instance?
- What is the author's family name? the title? keywords?
- Can a journal title abbreviation be used to search in this catalogue?
- What truncation symbols does this catalogue or database recognise?
- Will search-term truncation be a useful strategy?
- How do I interpret the results of my search?
- Is the item available in print or electronic format or both?
- Do I understand the arrangement of the library's collections?
- How do I ask the librarian for assistance—information desk or email or phone?
- What services are available if the library does not have my reference in stock?

Source: Dr D. Kingston, Information Services (Dentistry) Librarian, University of Sydney

Professional librarians are experts in information management. They represent a major resource for students; they can be extremely helpful partners in your learning. In many universities they offer classes to assist new students and advanced sessions for more senior groups. Even if you are confident of your library skills, it is well worth joining in such activities, as the world of information management is expanding and changing rapidly. University librarians may digitise important bibliographic resources, including required readings. They may place them on a secure university intranet or in a learning management system like WebCT, simplifying and streamlining access for students.

Recommended texts

When you start a new subject, your teachers will often offer guidance on the nature of the sources to be used for studying. They will usually provide a reading list for written assignments and indicate their expectations of the amount and depth of discussion required. Early in your health or social science studies, as you come to grips with new ideas and specialised terminologies, you will usually find textbooks to be a major resource. Good textbooks and educational CD-ROMs usually concentrate on summarising, interpreting, and explaining topics, perhaps including diagrams, models, and simplifications to help you understand complex ideas. If your university offers flexible e-learning, you may find that sections of textbooks or teachers' summaries are available on the local intranet. These will often assist you to understand key ideas.

As you progress, however, you will need to consult reviews or specialised books in which ideas from several sources are discussed and placed in a broader, often historical, context. These are secondary sources. In senior and honours years you are expected to consult primary sources (that is, the original written work of the experimenter(s) or the generator(s) of new ideas). While most teachers will continue to suggest appropriate reading, they will increasingly expect you to follow up interesting sources and locate your own information.

6.3   Library Pathfinder Questions 2: How to find some references on a *subject*

HANDY HINT

- Have I logically identified the main concepts in my research question?
- Do I need both books and journal articles on my topic?
- How do I find the best evidence?
- What other sorts of material will be useful?
- Which sources will be relevant to this topic?
- Will I start in the library catalogue or electronic databases?
- Do I need to consult the *Help* tools in each information source?
- Does this database have a controlled vocabulary to help me search systematically for my main concepts?
- Will textword searching be a useful strategy?
- Will textword truncation be a useful strategy?
- What truncation symbols does this catalogue or database recognise?
- Have I finished translating my concepts into search terms that can be used in this database?
- Do I need to review the use of Boolean terms to combine concepts logically?
- Have I logically combined my search terms?
- Have I logically combined my search statements?
- Should I narrow or expand my search?

Source: Dr D. Kingston, Information Services (Dentistry) Librarian, University of Sydney

Bibliographic catalogues and databases

Written materials in the health and social sciences are proliferating, so it is important to be able to locate relevant and useful sources of information efficiently. A library catalogue will help you to locate the book or journal you need to consult (provided that it is not misplaced on the wrong shelf and has not already been borrowed).

Many references are now stored in electronic bibliographic databases. These databases increase in number every year, along with the amount of information stored. Most libraries now provide electronic access to many library resources, and you are usually offered tutorial help (possibly online) in using them. Increasingly, too, you can read original articles from a journal electronically if you or your library has a subscription to the journal, and some journal volumes are posted free on the Internet a year or so after publication. You can arrange to print articles immediately, or view them on screen and make notes. As with photocopying, be selective in what you choose to print and save.

One obvious virtue of electronic databases of references is the power and ease of searching, achieved by storing key information in different 'fields'. Figure 6.1 shows typical fields for common sources (books, book chapters, and journal articles). The elements in brackets may or may not need to be included in your bibliography, depending on the system of referencing you are using.

Figure 6.1   Common fields in bibliographic databases

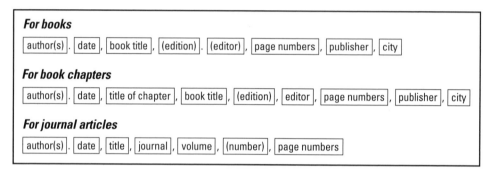

Many library databases allow you to search for words in one or more of the above fields, and often include a 'keyword' option. These features make it relatively straightforward to find references when you are starting a new search. In the following examples, the higlighted words can be placed in a field or used as keywords:

- 'Can I locate some recent articles on <u>myopia</u> in <u>school children</u>?'
- 'What are major <u>risk factors</u> for <u>colon cancer</u>?'

Progressively refine your search criteria if your search generates an overwhelming amount of data. For example, a search on *Medline* for 'risk factors and colon cancer since 1950' produced 52 items. Limiting the search to the last 10 years resulted in 39, and selecting 'human' and 'published in English' reduced the total to 33.

A second advantage of electronic databases is their capacity to save references directly to a disk or onto your computer. That is, instead of copying out the information by hand from the article (perhaps introducing errors), you can transfer the information electronically from the catalogue into your own computer. You may also be able to save and print an abstract.

The Internet

The Internet provides many and varied resources for the health and social sciences, but remember that few sites are checked for accuracy or quality. Be critical and selective when searching. You could check with your local librarian for sites that have been authenticated. At the end of this chapter we list a variety of websites that offer advice or tutorials on research strategies and on searching the Internet with increasing sophistication. Some Internet sites, such as open-access refereed journals and other resources provided by reputable universities, have been reviewed for quality and are reliable.

The two key databases for the health and medical sciences are *Medline* and *CINAHL*. You may also find it worthwhile to look at other general indexes such as *Sociofile* and *PsychInfo*, or specialist ones such as *Cancerlit*. Major resources of 'best evidence' are the *Cochrane Collaboration* <http://www.cochrane.org> for medical topics and the *Joanna Briggs Institute* <http://www.joannabriggs.edu.au/about/home.php> for the health and social sciences. These organisations conduct systematic reviews of articles on selected topics against agreed criteria, allowing health and social science professionals to identify the best evidence to inform their practice. Look at their websites to see if there has been a systematic review conducted on your topic of interest. This is not only good scholarship but it saves you a lot of time, as these are regarded as authoritative sources.

Increasingly, students are expected to keep a clear audit trail of their literature searches, and some teachers now require it. At the more advanced levels of study you may need to justify why you used particular keywords and how you used the databases for searching. An easy way to track what you have searched is to make use of keywords and keep the results of your searches. It may be useful to keep the information in a table. For example, in a search on shame and stigma in relation to lung cancer we could create a table like the one in Figure 6.2.

Figure 6.2   Example of a literature search audit table

Keywords CINAHL MEDLINE PsycINFO CANCERLitProQest Health/ MedicalProQuest Soc.Sc. & Humanities
Shame: 5291,0882900–2284,830
Guilt: 8283,9317,392–2915,505
Stigma: 1,6531,8472,5904812,678
Shame or guilt or stigma: 2,8206,46111,50820998210,000
Cancer: 38,843385,49911,541–10,00010,000
Cancer and shame or guilt or stigma: 328148150
Cancer and (shame or guilt): 1555
Cancer and stigma: 531
Lung cancer: 1,91025,44437226,023–4,718
Lung cancer and shame or guilt or stigma: 1335
Lung cancer and shame: 0
Lung cancer and (shame or guilt): 04
Lung cancer and stigma: 001
Guilt and lung cancer: 4

Advanced searching using a citation index

When reading an article or chapter, you can track *back* from its citations to find the original observation and the subsequent commentary of others. A citation index allows you to work *forward* in time.

A citation index lists authors whose work has been cited in any of a large range of journals and books. Importantly, it also provides information about where those papers and books have been referred to subsequently. Thus, working forward in time from a specific publication, you can identify authors who have cited the original article since it was published. It is then possible to track how a specific observation or idea has been developed and critiqued by others. The original observation may even have been refuted! Published writers can also measure the impact of their own work by consulting a citation index to see how often their original paper, book, or article has been referred to, and by whom. Using a citation index is particularly important if you are about to embark on a major investigation, such as a project in a senior year or in an honours or postgraduate program. Your search may prevent you from wasting time and resources by repeating research that has already effectively answered your question.

Databases of citations from published work exist for a number of disciplines. They are now extensive, especially for journal articles, less so for books. Annual and monthly lists are available. Major citation indexes include the *Sciences Citation Index* (SCI) and the *Social Sciences Citation Index* (SSCI).

Systematically recording, storing, and retrieving information

Keeping records

Because of the importance of written information for your studies and future practice, you should make a habit of systematically filing hard copies of information on topics that you are searching so that you can locate them again later. And when you file the data you collect you should also attach the exact and full details of the source of this information, firstly so that you can reference it properly and secondly so that if necessary you can find the reference again. (Referencing strategies are dealt with in Chapter 7.)

Although you may be tempted to photocopy all or many references identified by teachers, it is important to be selective. Read the article and decide whether it deserves to be copied in full or in part, or only noted for future reference. You may choose to summarise the important points, then save only the bibliographic information and perhaps an important figure or table or the list of references at the end. Photocopying whole chapters and articles does not commit them to memory, and you can rapidly accumulate so many that you cannot read them all. Nevertheless, particularly for a key assignment or a thesis, you may want the originals (or photocopies) beside you to ensure accuracy when you discuss specific points. If you cannot save an original document or a photocopy, you still need to make good notes and store them systematically so that they can be recovered easily. Folders, filing drawers, and boxes are convenient for keeping related hard copy together. If you label these containers carefully you should be able to retrieve the stored information efficiently and quickly.

Effective storage and retrieval of resources

Develop a simple, easily accessible system for storing your class notes and any photocopies, reference lists, and additional notes you have made. Sometimes your data will be in the form of hard copy (such as journal papers, computer printouts and newspaper cuttings); you may collect entire journal articles or summaries in hard copy. These data files would most likely be stored in a filing cabinet and listed alphabetically (by author or title) or chronologically (by date). You will probably need to develop an electronic storage system (e.g. for downloaded journal papers) alongside and cross-referenced with your hard-copy set.

If you are doing research, your data could be measurements or records of objects, human variables, or events. Such data could be recorded electronically or on paper and then transferred into a statistics package for analysis; Excel and SPSS are two such packages. Sometimes the data are in visual form, such as photographs or videotapes. Alternatively, you may be collecting qualitative data (e.g. via interviews), and you will need a system to manage the data from your tape recordings and the transcripts of these tapes. These may be filed according to the assigned code or pseudonym of your interviewee/research participant. You can make use of software such as Word, Annotape (for recording and playback), and Filemaker Pro for storage and voice-recognition tools for transcription.

Your database must be a system that works for you. It should allow you to label accurately (with full source/reference details) each piece of data, to store and retrieve items efficiently, and to proceed to the tasks of data analysis and report writing. Sometimes you will need to develop an indexing system, summary sheets, or cards by topic, to be able to cross-reference data stored systematically (e.g. alphabetically) with topics or sections of your assignment or thesis, and to cross-reference different data sets, such as electronic, hard copy, and media (e.g. tapes). When planning to write, you may want to rearrange these items temporarily by topic, so that you can collect all items relevant to one topic together while you write up that topic, but be sure to re-file them alphabetically to help you locate them easily in the future.

Further reading

Explore the sites listed below. They will provide assistance and offer ways of enhancing your skills in research and in searching the Web for relevant information.

Assistance, including tutorials

Abilock, D. 2002, 'Research', NUEVA Library Goal <http://nuevaschool.org/~debbie/library/research/research.html> accessed 15 March 2004.

About, Inc. 2004 <http://websearch.about.com/cs/howtosearch/index.htm> accessed 15 March 2004.

CSU Information Competence 1999, Online tutorials, Cal Poly State University, San Luis Obispo, California <http://www.lib.calpoly.edu/infocomp/modules/index.html> accessed 15 March 2004.

Horton, R. K. 2004, 'How to search the Internet: Searching and finding', P. L. Duffy Resource Centre, Trinity College, Western Australia <http://library.trinity.wa.edu.au/library/study/searching.htm> accessed 15 March 2004.

Learn the Net 2004, 'The animated Internet: How search engines work', Michael Lerner Productions <http://www.learnthenet.com/english/section/digdat.html> accessed 15 March 2004.

Library Online Tutorials 2003, 'How to do research on the Internet', Monash University. <http://www.lib.monash.edu.au/vl/www/wwwcon.htm> accessed 15 March 2004.

Notess, G. R. 2002, 'Basic Internet searching' <http://searchengineshowdown.com/strat/basic-search.html> accessed 15 March 2004.

University Libraries, University at Albany, State University of New York <http://library.albany.edu/internet/reference/learning.html> accessed 15 March 2004.

University of Florida Information skills mini-course, 'Lesson 6: Research strategies' <http://web.uflib.ufl.edu/instruct2/mini/intro6.html> accessed 15 March 2004.

USC Beaufort Library 2004, 'Bare bones 101: A basic turorial on searching the Web', USC Beaufort. <http://www.sc.edu/beaufort/library/pages/bones.html> accessed 3 June 2004.

Seeking new strategies

UC Berkeley Library 2004, 'Finding information on the Internet: A tutorial', University of California <http://www.lib.berkeley.edu/TeachingLib/Guides/Internet/FindInfo.html> accessed 15 March 2004.

Best strategies matched to search

Abilock, D. 2004, 'Information literacy: Search strategies', Noodle Tools. <http://www.noodletools.com/debbie/literacies/information/5locate/adviceengine.html> accessed 15 March 2004.

Strategies by discipline

Internet Navigator Online Course 2003, University of Utah <http://medstat.med.utah.edu/navigator/about.htm> accessed 15 March 2004.

RDN Virtual Training Suite 2004, University of Bristol <http://www.vts.rdn.ac.uk/> accessed 15 March 2004.

Systematic reviews

Cochrane: The Reliable Source of Evidence in Healthcare 2004, The Cochrane Collaboration <http://www.cochrane.org/> accessed 15 March 2004.

REFERENCING AND MANAGING REFERENCES

Joy Higgs, Joan Rosenthal, and Ann Sefton

KEY TOPICS

→ The place of referencing in scholarly writing

→ How to reference

→ Referencing strategies: which, when, how, why to use, how much

Introduction

Referencing is about honesty, acknowledgment, legitimation, and accuracy. It is an essential component of authentic and high quality scholarly writing. Scholarly or informal writing may be wholly original, in which case the author is the only source listed. In most cases, however, written, verbal, and electronic text is built on ideas and arguments that other people have already expressed. It is honest and responsible to acknowledge the authors of these existing ideas by referencing their publications or communications in your work.

Referencing and sources

References acknowledge the sources of the ideas, information, data, and arguments you present in your work. There are two main types of source (Spatt 1983, p. 353). A *primary source* is a work that gives you direct or primary knowledge of the event, period, or original thought. It is often an article written about the findings of research or an educational/information/clinical strategy. Primary sources also include health policy documents, medical records, case notes, and the aggregated information from national censuses and bureaus of statistics. Writers talking or writing about their first-hand experiences also fit into this category.

A *secondary source* provides commentary written after and about a primary source. Secondary sources are valuable when they summarise, critique, or comment upon a range of primary sources. They can save you a great deal of time finding or reading all the original works, particularly if those works are difficult to obtain (e.g. unpublished manuscripts and very old publications). However, your work, particularly research work and theses, needs to demonstrate your original ideas and insights, your critiques and your interpretations of primary sources; so don't rely too heavily on secondary sources. Particularly in postgraduate research work, primary sources should predominate.

If you are the source of an idea or argument, you have two broad ways of indicating this:

- implicitly; if no source is explicitly indicated then the author of the essay, thesis, article, etc., is assumed to be the source. All the arguments you present will be attributed to you.
- explicitly, using the first person (e.g. 'I have found that …'; 'In my opinion …') or using the third person (e.g. 'It can be argued that …'; 'There are many ways of interpreting these data; for example, …'). Note that the use of the first person in academic writing is not acceptable in some schools and disciplines.

The importance of referencing style and conventions

The style of referencing used in scholarly writing and the referencing conventions (expectations, systems, etc.) are influenced by the requirements of the writing situation—the referencing system used by your institution, school or teacher; the expectations of your field (e.g. medicine or psychology); the journal or publisher (see the 'guide to contributors' information in journals); and your own preferences.

For assignments, you may be required to format the references according to a particular departmental style, often based on a key book or journal in that discipline. Copy the required style exactly. If you have any questions, ask your lecturer *before* you start formatting. If there are no specific requirements, choose a well-known referencing style and use it consistently.

HANDY HINT ☞ 7.1 Following referencing guidelines

Referencing correctly is one of the important skills you learn when you learn to write. Most tertiary institutions have their own referencing guidelines. Follow the instructions in these guidelines carefully.

Bibliographies and reference lists

All the references that you have used in a paper or thesis must be included in your reference list at the end. Alternatively, if your arguments have been indirectly influenced by a range of readings and you want to acknowledge all of them, even if you haven't referred to them directly, you can include them in a second list called a bibliography. Check with your lecturer before handing in a bibliography, as this practice is not always acceptable. It is often assumed that the breadth of your reading will be evident in the way you construct your argument. The references in a bibliography or reference list are usually listed alphabetically.

Major referencing systems

Three common methods for referencing in the health and social professions are the Harvard system, the APA (American Psychological Association) system, and the Vancouver system.

The Harvard and APA systems use the *author, year* format in the text. The Vancouver, or numerical, referencing system uses superscripted numbers to designate references in the text (e.g. 'The following major studies[1–3] involved …') and lists the references in numerical sequence in the reference list (see Hay et al. 2002, p. 149). Some journals require the same reference to be assigned the same number on each occasion in the text (which entails manual insertion of the superscripted number), so that the reference list contains each reference only once. You can find detailed instructions on how to use these systems in many places: see Handy Hint 7.2.

7.2 Resources on referencing

Harvard referencing system

Note that different versions of the Harvard system exist. Two of these are detailed in the following two references.

Murdoch University Library 2004, 'How to cite references: Author date style' <http://wwwlib.murdoch.edu.au/guides/citation/authordate.html> accessed 25 March 2004. This version of the Harvard system is based on the American *Chicago Manual of Style*.
Style Manual for Authors, Editors and Printers, 2002, 6th edn, rev. by Snooks & Co., John Wiley & Sons Australia.

APA referencing system

American Psychological Association 2001, *Publication Manual of the American Psychological Association*, 5th edn, American Psychological Association, Washington, DC.
APA Online 2004 <http://www.apastyle.org/> accessed 25 March 2004.

Vancouver system

National Library of Medicine 2003 <http://www.nlm.nih.gov/bsd/uniform_requirements.html> accessed 25 March 2004.

Additional sources

Digital Information Services Center 2003 <http://www.researchsoftware.nl/links/Citation_Guides/more2.html> accessed 12 November 2003. Web-based sources of some useful information on citation.
Capital Community College Library 2004, 'A guide for writing research papers based on Modern Language Association (MLA) documentation' <http://webster.commnet.edu/mla/index.shtml> accessed 12 November 2003. A Web-based resource on writing generally, but with help on citation.
Lee, I. 2004, 'A research guide for students' <http://www.aresearchguide.com/styleguides.html> accessed 12 November 2003. A Web-based guide to citations and outlines of the requirements for some common publishers' or journal styles.

HANDY HINT

Examples of references using the Harvard system

In-text references

References in the text are written as follows:

- Single reference, 1-2 authors: '(Jackson 2000)' or 'Jackson (2000) argued that …'. Note that the reference comes before the full stop if it is at the end of the sentence.
- Single reference, more than 2 authors: '(Jackson et al. 2000)'. However, if this abbreviated format does not differentiate multi-authored references that were published in the same year, include as many authors as are needed to identify the reference, e.g. '(Jackson, Black et al. 2000)' contrasts with '(Jackson, Morton et al. 2000)'.
- Multiple references: list these in alphabetical order (unless directed otherwise, say by a journal's style guide or by lecturers, who may require the references to be in chronological order).
- Quotes: include page numbers as described below. The page number may be stated as part of the reference, as in '(Wentworth 2001, p. 96)', or located at the end of a block quote.
- Personal communications: '(Arrilla June 2002, personal communication)'. Occasionally your source is not published. You may have had a conversation with someone. This is called a personal communication. It does not need to be included in the reference list.

References in the reference list or bibliography

Journal articles

Holmes, C. A. 1990, 'Alternatives to natural science foundations for nursing', *International Journal of Nursing Studies*, vol. 27, pp. 187–98.

Edited books

Basmajian, J. V. & Banerjee, S. N. (eds) 1996, *Clinical Decision Making in Rehabilitation*, Churchill Livingstone, New York.

Authored books

Gilligan, C. 1982, *In a Different Voice: Psychological Theory and Women's Development*, Harvard University Press, Cambridge, Massachusetts.

Book chapters

Giltrow, J. & Valiquette, M. 1994, 'Genres and knowledge: Students writing in the disciplines', in *Learning and Teaching Genre*, eds A. Freedman & P. Medway, Heinemann/Boynton Cook, Portsmouth, New Hampshire, pp. 47–62.

Web publications

Websites change over time. They may even disappear! To clearly reference and give credibility to a Web-based reference, include the date you accessed it as well as the URL:

National Health Service 2000, 'Meeting the challenge: A strategy for the allied health professions', NHS. Available at <www.doh.gov.uk/meetingthechallenge> accessed 15 November 2001.

Lectures and lecture notes

You may want to quote or refer to information gleaned from notes you took or notes that were provided at a lecture you attended. If this information was also published, cite it in the same way as a published reference. If it was not published, provide the name of the course and the year:

Communication Studies 301, 2000, lecture notes.

Newspaper and magazine articles

If the author is named in a byline in a newspaper or magazine article, write the reference in the same way as for a journal article, but stating the date of publication instead of the volume number. If no author's name is provided, use the name of the newspaper or magazine:

The Australian, 15 June 2003, 'Where are they now?', p. 25.

Quotations

Quotations are verbatim extracts from published material, extracts from research data transcripts (e.g. interviews), or verbal communications. In each case you are citing an author's opinion, information, perspectives, etc., about the topic you are discussing; therefore you must attribute this material to the original author/source. This is done by referencing the source and including the page number (if published), transcript reference (if research data) or date (if verbal information) pertaining to the quote. Don't overdo quotes. Remember that it's your ideas and critique that need to be presented, not just other people's ideas. Here are some guidelines for formatting and reporting quotes:

- Use inverted commas for quotes; for example, 'The incidence of influenza in this population rose to 13% in the subsequent two years' (Francis 1976, p. 42). (Note that the reference is within the sentence, before the full stop.)
- Use double inverted commas for quotes within quotes, that is, when the original author was using quotation marks already. For example, 'Review of the various reports led to the conclusion that there had been "a significant mis-representation" of the findings in several cases' (Kennedy 1998, p. 339).
- For large quotes (more than 5 lines), use a left-indented paragraph. No inverted commas are used. For example:

    > Although clinicians may have knowledge of 'best practice', according to professional standards or the literature for a particular condition, they recognise that such generic best practice might not be the most appropriate for a particular patient's context, or best according to that patient's own perspective and priorities. (Trede & Higgs 2003, p. 67)

- Omit words from a quotation if you think some words are unnecessary to your discussion and their omission would not change the original author's meaning. Use an ellipsis (…) to indicate that words have been deleted. Note that there is a space before and after the three dots.
- Add words if necessary to make sense of the quotation (e.g. to explain words like 'it' and 'they') or to maintain the flow of the text where you have inserted the quotation. Put square brackets around the added words. For example, 'For many patients this [increased waiting time] was a major problem.'
- If the text you are quoting contains inaccurate or undesirable spelling, words, or grammar, you may insert '(sic)' in the quote to show that you note the inaccuracy but you are quoting correctly from the original. For example, 'Practitioners who are in a sole practice needs (sic) to develop networking skills …'
- If desired, you may add emphasis within a quotation by italicising a word or words. Then write '[emphasis added]' after the quote.

Specific referencing strategies and tools

The following points explain some of the finer details of referencing:

- **Referencing in drafts.** The most common general method of referencing is by author and year (and page number if required). Use this method when writing so that you can reference accurately, even if you later have to change to another method such as superscripted numbers.
- **a and b references.** You may be referencing two papers by Smith and Hauser, both published in 2001. In this case you need first to ensure that when you are making notes from those papers, and when you are writing about them, you keep note of which paper you are referring to at each point. Second, list the references in the reference list as '(a)'

and '(b)', using the authors and title alphabetically (ignore 'a', 'the' etc) to determine the (a) and (b) ordering. In your paper refer to the sources as 'Smith and Hauser (2001a)' and 'Smith and Hauser (2001b)' consistently throughout the text. For example:

> Smith, R. E. & Hauser, L. S. 2001a, *Researching Lived Experiences*, Smithson Press, Cambridge.

> Smith, R. E. & Hauser, L. S. 2001b, *Textual Analysis*, Perrington Books, Chicago.

- **et al.** (*et alia*). This literally means 'and other persons' (Peters 1995, p. 254). The use of 'et al.' saves the reader having to read many authors' names and possibly lose the flow of the text. If you have used 'et al.' in the text be sure that the reader can determine exactly which reference you are referring to in the list. Instructions for using 'et al.' vary, and you should follow the requirements of the system you are using. (For instance, some systems require all authors to be listed on the first mention of a reference in the text.) We recommend using 'et al.' (throughout the text) for references with more than two authors unless your local system/instructions require otherwise.
- **ibid.** 'This referencing device is an abbreviated form of the Latin *ibidem* meaning "in the same place". Used in follow-up references to a particular book, chapter, or page, it directs readers to the same source or place as was mentioned in the immediately preceding reference. It substitutes the author's name, the title of the book or article, and as much of what follows as would be identical.' (Peters 1995, p. 360). For example:

> Bridge and Karim (2002) reported that among the 240 first year students, 70% had their own car. It seems that this sample may have been rather affluent. Among the 195 third year students, 60% lived away from home (ibid.).

- **op cit.** 'This Latin abbreviation is *only* used in footnotes and endnotes, as a follow-up to the previous reference. It means "in the work (already) cited". It saves the writer having to repeat the full title of the work referred to, provided it had been cited in full in an earlier footnote … However the use of op. cit. is declining (and being actively discouraged by some publishers such as the Chicago University Press).' (Peters 1995, p. 543).
- **Page numbers.** In the text you must use page number(s) when quoting (see the Peters example immediately above). Some disciplines and institutions also require you to include the page number in your reference in the text when you are referring to a key idea or information from the reference, even if you are not directly quoting. Check your local rules or publication guidelines.
- **Paraphrasing.** You paraphrase when you are using an idea or data from a source but are not quoting it directly; for example, when the section is extensive and you want to abbreviate it, or to avoid excessive quotations. Paraphrases should be referenced the same as any idea derived from another source. Page numbers may be included but are not essential unless your local convention/system requires them.
- **Describing your own work.** There are times when you are describing your research activities and you need to reference some aspect, such as the method used. Remember that the author of the work you are referencing did not write about your work. It is incorrect to write:

> I used a reflective practitioner approach to the focus groups (Schön 1983).

Instead, you should clearly indicate what it was that the author referred to actually wrote about, and what you are writing about yourself. Ways of doing this include the following:

Based upon the in-depth interview strategies discussed by Minichiello et al. (1995), I developed an interview schedule to use with my participants.

I utilised Schön's (1983) notion of 'the reflective practitioner' to frame the focus-group discussion.

I used a grounded-theory approach (based on Strauss & Corbin 1990).

My research utilised a phenomenology of practice strategy (*qua* van Manen 1996). ('*qua*' here means 'as in').

- **Citations.** Sometimes you are using a secondary source and the author refers directly to a work by another person. The format for reporting this is as follows:

   Example 1: (Johns 2000, p. 225, citing Graveney 1982).

In this case, Johns mentioned Graveney but did not provide the reference details. In your references, list Johns only.

   Example 2: (Graveney 1982, p. 84, cited in Blakehurst 2001, p. 21).

In this case, Blakehurst quoted from Graveney and provided the full reference details. In your references, list Graveney and give details of both the Graveney and Blakehurst publications within that reference.

Developing and storing your own reference lists

When developing a system for storing your references you must record enough information for you to be able to report the reference (and relevant content) accurately later and if needed track down the references again. It is frustrating knowing that you have read some important information on your topic somewhere, but don't have enough bibliographical detail to locate it. Having comprehensive bibliographical data may also allow you to retrieve references when you have only a limited recall of important components (such as 'that useful Canadian article published last year I read on muscular dystrophy …' or 'which of L. Q. Smith's nursing papers referred to renal failure?'). Be selective in storing data. For a writing task, you may have a long list of sources but only some will turn out to be useful. Store permanently only those that you have actually read and cited, or might want to consult in future. Don't spend more time making your database than you do writing your essay! Remember to back up your electronic reference database. Keep at least one copy away from the main computer, on disk, CD, or server. Relying on a single reference database on one machine puts you in danger from damage, theft, breakdown, or power failure: you could lose years of work.

Electronic reference-management systems

The best bibliographic reference-management systems are electronic, because of their convenience in storing data and relative ease of searching through data. The reference database(s) you develop will be invaluable in future professional life and will support publication of your work. Because such management systems offer so many features, they are not necessarily easy to use, but it is worthwhile persevering! There are many advantages in using electronic reference-management systems. Once the information is entered accurately, it need never be retyped. Electronic references inserted into your paper, essay, or thesis ensure that citations in the text will match the list of references at the end (i.e. all the references will be listed and all names and years will be correct, as long as you took the trouble to type them in accurately in the first place). This saves a great deal of checking time, particularly for theses.

Purpose-written bibliographic programs include EndNote, ProCite, and Reference Manager. Each entry has a unique sequential identifying number, specific to that database. If that reference is copied into another database, it is assigned a different number. It is ideal to own your reference database program, but they can be expensive, even with academic pricing. Ownership gives you a manual (essential reading) and access to help, information, and upgrades, and you can take it into professional life. If you cannot afford to purchase a copy, your university may have a license to offer student access on university-owned machines or a local network. If you plan to purchase, choose a reliable program used in your institution. You will then have access to training and advice from librarians, staff, and senior students, and manuals or a help desk may be available. Many library sites provide online guidance. Be warned that the major programs are powerful, but complex; they have individual quirks, so you will need practice. Start using them early, before you meet the pressures of senior courses. Everyone needs the manual (or a guide) at the stage of formatting.

Principles of storing references

Enough information should be stored to allow you to access and cite a specific work, without ambiguity. References are stored electronically in 'fields' that can be searched independently.

The number and types of fields you need to include in your references vary among disciplines. Check the journals in your area of study and your university's referencing guide. Lists of references must be specific and accurate, to ensure academic honesty and promote efficiency in locating sources. Record the locations (e.g. in the library) and reference numbers of hard copies in libraries and other locations. The basic principles of referencing are straightforward, but complexity arises in part from the different conventions used in different publications. Publishers or editors determine the sequence of the fields and demand specific formatting (regarding the use of bold type, italics, punctuation, spacing, etc.). Bibliographic packages allow you to format your references in a number of different styles.

Organising your reference database: keywords

Whatever storage system you choose, you must know which fields are needed regularly, so that you can retrieve and cite articles accurately. It is useful to store additional information by adding keywords (e.g. physical location of a source, important issues not included in the title), even if you are maintaining a paper-based system. Many published articles stored in electronic databases have keywords included to aid searching. Be systematic in developing your own keyword systems. Here are some examples:

- **for science:** topic, issue, or discipline; experimental strategy; body system, organ, and/or region; original paper or review; issues specific to your interests; location of source;
- **for clinical studies:** topic, discipline, and/or diagnosis; nature/type of study; issue of concern; original paper or review; issues specific to your interests; location of source.

You can download references (including abstracts) from an electronic bibliographic database without having to do any retyping. That is, while searching the library's database(s), you can select references to add to your own electronic list if you have the software set up correctly. In most cases, the references will transfer seamlessly, but each system is different so you will need some local training and assistance from librarians.

Groups of students may share the task of entering information into a joint database, while each individual student can make use of the stored data. The downside of using a database that others have helped to create is that you can only locate and retrieve the information if it was entered correctly. Accuracy and completeness of the data entry are essential. You will need to proofread your database regularly to identify missing data and duplicate entries.

Even if the transfer from electronic sources cannot be automated, a 'cut and paste' approach still saves some time and reduces copying errors. With this approach, you highlight/select and copy the contents of each field displayed in the source file and then paste it into the relevant field of your own database.

You can store all your references in one large file, or develop more than one file if you want to store different categories of literature that do not generally overlap (e.g. basic science, clinical research, evidence-based practice, and practice management). It is often helpful to develop a specific database reference library for each writing project. Written work can then be saved together with its own reference library in a folder. You have to be careful and systematic, since the number of each reference is unique to the specific library database. When ready for formatting, the in-text citations are replaced by a number, or by a citation with the name(s) and date. Each in-text reference will be matched precisely with an item in the bibliography.

Developing a set of references as you write an assignment, thesis or paper

When writing, open both the word processing file and the master reference database, often called a *library* in reference programs. To insert a citation into your text, toggle to the database, select one or more references that you want to insert in the text, copy them, return to the word processing file, and paste. Citations then appear, each with a unique identifier in the text, as set out in Figure 7.1. Once the writing is completed you remove these bibliographic identifiers, to leave just the required reference details (e.g. author/s, year, page number if quote) in the text. (See your software program for full instructions.)

Figure 7.1   Writing and inserting references by highlighting, cutting, and pasting: An example

---

Step 1: Selecting the reference(s) from the database
In your database, the references you want might look like those listed below. Highlight the one(s) you want to use (here 5 have been selected) to support a point or an argument you have just made, then cut the highlighted references:

Abraham	1995	Australian health trends
Adelstein	1994	Searching
Agan	1987	Intuitive knowing as a dimension of nursing
Aiken	1988	The problem of nonresponse in survey research
Albanese	2000	The decline and fall of humanism in medical education
Arnold	2002	Assessing professional behaviour: yesterday, today, and tomorrow
Bashford	1998	Purity and pollution
Bates	1997	Restructuring the university for technological change
Battles	2001	A system of analysing medical errors to improve GME

Step 2: Pasting into the text
Return to your text and paste them in. When you insert references from EndNote, they look like this in the text:

[Agan 1987 #33; Battles 2001 #37; Adelstein 1994 #32; Battles 1997 #1486; Bashford 1998 #34].

The numbers refer to the unique number of that reference in your database.

Step 3: Formatting the references
The examples below indicate how the citations might look in the text after you have completed your work and formatted the text:

Example (a): (Agan 1987; Aiken 1988; Adelstein et al. 1994; Bashford 1998; Battles and Shea 2001)
Example (b): (1–5), which will match the numbered list of references at the end.

Step 4: Creating a list of references
At the same time, a reference list will be formatted automatically at the end of the article, with the style depending on the format you choose:

Example (a):
Adelstein, S. J., S. T. Carver, H. Goldman and M.B. Ramos (1994). Transitional organization. *New Pathways to Medical Education.* D. C. Tosteson, S. J. Adelstein and S. T. Carver. Boston, MA, Harvard University Press: 139–57.
Agan, R. D. (1987). 'Intuitive knowing as a dimension of nursing.' *Advances in Nursing Science* **10**: 63–70.
Aiken, L. R. (1988). 'The problem of nonresponse in survey research.' *Journal of Experimental Education* **56**: 116–19.
Bashford, A. (1998). *Purity and Pollution.* London, Methuen.
Battles, J. B. and C. E. Shea (2001). 'A system of analyzing medical errors to improve GME curricula and programs.' *Academic Medicine* **76**(2): 125–33.
Example (b):
A similar list in full, but each is allocated a unique number to match the number in the text.

Note that the requirements of an assignment may include instructions on how to set out the references. For example, rather than formatting as in 4(a) above, you may be expected to use bold or plain text, or to underline the titles; the order of items in references may change; journal names may be abbreviated; or the sequence of the authors' names and initials could be different. Carefully read the instructions from your teacher or your targeted publication, and make sure you follow them.

Formatting references for a writing task

There is an extensive library of publishers' formats available within reference software programs, which can simplify the task of formatting your references. Occasionally you have to select formatting that is quite similar to the required referencing style, then create your own style, although a search of the reference program's website may yield an appropriate match.

Leave yourself enough time for this formatting component of your task. Even with training and experience, people frequently need to consult the relevant manual and may need to resort to trial and error. Be sure to proofread and spell-check the reference list at the end of the process and go back to correct any errors in your database. If you are citing from British, American, and Australian books and journals, you will find variations in spelling within the references (e.g. in the titles of book, articles, and journals); these should always be left as published.

References from the same database can readily be formatted for different purposes. Then if one journal rejects your manuscript, you can quickly change its referencing style to follow the bibliographic conventions of a different journal.

Other electronic reference-storage systems

General computer-based filing systems (e.g. Filemaker Pro and Excel) can be used to store references electronically, but they lack the flexibility, versatility, and power of the purpose-designed bibliographic programs. Cutting and pasting electronically saves time when entering references into your own database and when assembling citations and references for written work. Formatting the items in a reference list manually takes great concentration, skill, and an eye for detail; it is less efficient than using a bibliographic program. A spreadsheet (e.g. Excel) can be set up to store references in cells horizontally across the page, with each vertical column dedicated to a specific field, and notes can be added in additional columns. Word processing programs, such as Word and WordPerfect, can also be used to create searchable tables or lists of references. With all the above systems, storage is secure and the database can be searched, but even with the cut-and-paste tool it is time-consuming to put references into the text and to format the reference list.

Hard-copy reference-management systems

If you do not have reliable access to a computer, you can use system cards that can be sorted in different ways to store and manage your references. Indeed, cards (or printouts of your electronic reference list) are convenient when you are in the library reading books and journals, even if you intend to transfer the information later to an electronic system. They allow you to check quickly whether you have already copied that article. If a card file is your major resource, remember to store *all* the information needed to identify the unique article, book, or journal. It is also particularly helpful to have a structured keyword system (as described

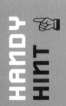

7.3 Managing references

- Accurately note information on all useful articles, books, and chapters that you read.
- Develop your own storage system for references.
- Learn to use an electronic reference database as early as you can.
- Ensure that you record enough fields to relocate and cite the reference. Include the library and library catalogue number (or other source), in case you have to find the original item again.
- Download references electronically when possible, to avoid retyping and potentially introducing errors.
- Back up all data regularly and store a copy away from your computer.

HANDY HINT

above). A master file-card can be prepared to remind you of all the information needed. Further, you should record the original location or library reference number, and make a note of where you have stored a photocopy or abstract. If you want to keep references from different subject areas separate, you can use different sets of card files. And remember that even with a paper- or card-based system you should back it up (e.g. by photocopying) and store it safely!

Conclusion

Referencing has two main purposes: it demonstrates the academic honesty of your writing and informs readers of the sources of your ideas and information. If your readers want to follow up on any of the sources you mention, they should be able to obtain all the details they need, from your writing, to track down any published background material.

This entails a great deal of care on your part. First, you must take care to note down all the details of sources that you consult, so you can provide these details (page numbers, publication information, etc.) if you eventually refer to the sources in your writing. Second, you must take care to acknowledge and record accurately any sources that have contributed to what you write.

References

Note: Some references in this chapter have been included for illustrative purposes only. They are not included in this reference list.

Hay, I., Bochner, D. & Dungey, C. 2002, *Making the Grade: A Guide to Successful Communication and Study*, Oxford University Press, Melbourne.

Peters, P. 1995. *The Cambridge Australian English Style Guide*, Cambridge University Press, Melbourne.

Style Manual for Authors, Editors and Printers 2002, 6th edn, rev. by Snooks & Co., John Wiley & Sons Australia.

Spatt, B. 1983, *Writing from Sources*, St Martin's Press, New York.

Teitelbaum, H. 1982, *How to Write a Thesis: A Guide to the Research Paper*, Monarch Press, New York.

Useful resources

Software

Note: You need to check the compatibility of versions of the software with the computer platform, the version and type of operating system, and the version of the word processor you use.

EndNote <http://www.endnote.com/> accessed 11 November 2003. Versions for Windows and Mac.

Reference Manager <http://www.refman.com/> accessed 11 November 2003. Windows only.

ProCite <http://www.procite.com/> accessed 11 November 2003. Versions for Windows and Mac (the latter with fewer options).

WriteNote. This is a recent Web-based tool for student research and writing; it may become available at your institution. For some information go to http://www.researchsoftware.nl/links/net and type 'writenote' into the search box.

08 WRITING JOURNAL PAPERS

Annette Street and Joy Higgs

KEY TOPICS

→ Choosing the right journal

→ Writing a plan

→ Designing the paper

→ Editing and revising

→ Preparation for submission

→ Responding to reviewers

Introduction

A journal article is the most common form of international communication about scholarly work in the health and social sciences. Articles take a variety of forms and cover a range of interests, from editorials, opinion pieces, research papers, debates, and systematic reviews to papers describing innovations in health education and practice. Journals are targeted to selected audiences and have specific conventions about how material is presented. Choosing the right journal and preparing your article to be acceptable to that journal are important skills. You will usually have a supervisor or other member of staff who can offer advice (and who may be a co-author).

Choosing the right journal

It is a waste of time to write an article and *then* try to find a journal that will accept it. As soon as you have a draft of your ideas, begin to search for the right journal. Ask yourself the following questions: What is the purpose of this paper? What type of message or research am I writing about? Who is my audience? There needs to be a clear match between the audience of the journal and the audience of your paper. If your topic is specific to a select audience, compose a list of journals that publish in that area. A paper entitled 'Sharing responsibility in home birth practice' would fit in midwifery, health-sociology, or women's health journals. Your article may be appropriate to a broader multidisciplinary health- and social-science audience. For example, 'Seasonal versus perennial allergic rhinitis: Patterns of use of drugs and medical resources' would be a topic of interest to a range of health professionals caring for people with asthma.

Once you have considered the potential audience for your article and matched it to a list of possible journals, do your homework on the journals. Peer-reviewed journals are journals that send each prospective article to selected reviewers to judge its quality and its compatibility with the journal's aims, and to give advice on how to the paper could be improved. These journals are valued because the review process ensures that every article has been validated by experts before it is published. Read carefully the 'information to contributors' provided by the journal (usually inside the cover or on the journal's website). Also read the table of contents of some past issues. These can often be found online or in your university or hospital library. Knowing what has been published recently is helpful, as some journals try to get a mix of topics and others will accept further articles on a topic as long as they have a different angle or important new information. If you are not sure if the journal will be interested in your topic, you (or your supervisor) can email the editor to ask if a submission on your topic would be considered. The editor may alert you to the fact that they have other articles on this topic ready for publication and may want yours to be considered for a series, or may tell you that they are not looking for more articles of this type or that it doesn't match the journal audience's needs. This helps you make a decision without wasting your time sending it to a journal that is not interested. By doing your homework in advance, you could save yourself a great deal of time preparing and formatting the paper particularly for that journal, and waiting possibly many months to receive feedback from reviewers who ultimately recommend rejecting the paper. Questions to consider in this analysis are included in Handy Hint 8.1.

HANDY HINT ☞ **8.1 Choosing a journal**

- What are the journal's aims and scope?
- Does my paper fit with them?
- What kinds of article are published in this journal?
- Who is the main journal audience?
- Is the journal published internationally?
- What is the standing of the journal?
- How long are the articles in the journal?
- What referencing style does this journal use?

It is also helpful to look at the style of writing that is accepted by the proposed journal. By looking at other papers you can see, for instance, whether writing in the first person or in a narrative style is accepted, or whether a more technical or scientific language is required. If your paper is a literature review, make sure the selected journal accepts literature reviews for publication. You need to consider the structure of papers of a similar genre to yours that have been published. For example, you may want to describe the findings of a survey. Check how surveys are generally reported (Fink 2002) and see how they are presented in the journal. Look to see if a journal predominantly publishes research papers, and whether they include qualitative or quantitative research or both. Remember that different research approaches are written up quite differently (see, for example, Llewellyn 1996; Peat et al. 2002; Smith 1998).

8.2   Review past issues of a journal

- What topics have been covered recently?
- Is my topic similar to other recent papers and compatible with the journal's goals and style?
- Does the journal have a student section?
- What styles of article are accepted: experimental work? literature reviews? systematic reviews? methodological articles? opinion pieces? case studies?

HANDY HINT

Take into account whether the journal's articles have a separate introduction, background, and literature review, or whether these sections are combined or not required. Look at the number of words generally allocated to each section, to guide the structure of your paper. For example, you may want to know if the journal accepts articles with quotes from research interviews or clinical observations. Or you may need to know how many tables or figures the journal accepts in an article. In any case, don't include unnecessary tables, figures, or inserts; reviewers will reject them.

Writing plan

Once you have chosen your journal it is a good idea to start with a writing plan. Collect a couple of articles that have been structured like the one you are planning to write (not on the same topic). If you intend to write a theoretical argument then choose theoretical papers that are structured using literature. If you have conducted a research project then you need to find a paper that matches the style of research that you have done (see Peat et al. 2002; Sandler 2003). Then think of each paper as a template for your own. Using this template you can make a plan of the sequence of sections and determine how detailed or how long each needs to be (see Handy Hint 8.3, p. 76). The plan should reflect the interests of the journal, whether it is science-based, social-science/humanities-based, or education-based, or accepts papers from a range of traditions.

Writing with colleagues

It is a common practice in the health and social sciences to write with one's colleagues, particularly when writing up collaborative research or a joint theoretical paper. Collaborative writing has the potential to produce a richer paper, on the principle that two or more heads are better than one. It does, however, add to the preparation time, as it requires considerable ongoing negotiation if it is to work well. If you are planning to do a joint paper, you need to be clear at the outset about what contribution each person will make to the paper. One person might contribute expertise in the methods whereas another may have specific professional knowledge. Some journals ask that you give a percentage weighting for the

HANDY HINT ☞ **8.3 Sample writing plan**

Journal paper

- Total words allowed: 3000
- Title (no more than ten words)
- Abstract (no more than 200 words)
- Keywords (up to 5)
- Reference style: Vancouver

Body of paper

- Introduction (about 500 words)—includes rationale, study aims, and key literature; justifies the need for and explains the scope of the paper.
- Method (about 500 words)—includes sample/participants, data-collection methods, data-analysis strategies, and ethics.
- Results/findings (750 words plus up to four tables or figures)—answers the research question or provides the evidence supporting your argument.
- Discussion (800–900 words)—analyses the findings in relation to the topic and the supporting literature.
- Conclusion, limitations, recommendations—reiterate new knowledge, outline limitations of the paper, and make recommendations for further action.

contribution of each person (Watts & Jackson 1998) when you submit a joint paper. This requirement is also used in university reporting of publications to national funding bodies. You must also be clear on who the first-listed and subsequent authors will be, and who will take responsibility for ensuring that the paper meets the standards of the target journal and for submitting the final agreed version. This person will usually be the contact person, whose institutional address appears with the paper and who will deal with correspondence with the journal editor.

Designing the paper

When you choose a title, make sure it uses relevant keywords, so that other people will be able to quickly find your article in their searches. Creative, eye-catching titles need a subtitle that clarifies the topic and method. Sometimes a well-crafted abstract will be the guide for the paper, but always return to it at the end of writing the paper to make sure it reflects the content and logic of the final draft. 'Keywords' are sometimes also requested; it is important to choose ones that fit with the choices in major search engines. You can find these in online databases such as Medline, CINAHL, and Sociofile.

When you begin to plan for the body of the paper, remember that journals are interested in new information. Organise your material to focus on the knowledge that you are adding to what is known, rather than try to cover everything that can be said on the topic. Select and order your material to develop a strong argument (Greenwood 1998). It is often helpful to develop a framework or outline to indicate the logic of your argument and the flow of the paper.

Keep accurate records of sources as you write. Decide which sources you will quote directly and which you will paraphrase; both types of inclusion in the text will need to be referenced. Be cautious and limit the use of direct quotations, and summarise key conclusions that you want to support or refute. Remember it is your work you are presenting; don't just regurgitate other people's work. Make sure you understand exactly what constitutes plagiarism and avoid deliberately or accidentally plagiarising other people's work (see Chapter 3). Set up your referencing system. It is usually considered good scholarship to acknowledge the first author(s) who generated a new idea or conclusion. Otherwise, use up-to-date references unless you have a good reason for using earlier work. Explain why you are drawing on earlier work. Choose the data (e.g. quotes, tables, and graphics) you want to include to support your argument or explain your findings, and consider the best format for presentation.

Then write a draft of the whole paper. Make sure that you discuss the scope and limitations of the paper, so that readers know what to expect as they read it (see Pirkis & Gardner 1998). Remember to critically review, not just retell, the literature. The literature review needs to provide sufficient background to locate your work in its context.

Good writing is clear and logical. Don't use technical jargon unnecessarily. Always introduce and define complex or technical language that would not be familiar to your readers. This will depend on whether you have chosen a specialist journal or a more general one. You can use commonly accepted acronyms (e.g. 'WHO' for the World Health Organization), but if the acronym (or an abbreviation you develop yourself, such as 'ECS' for Extended Community Support) is less common or likely to be unfamiliar to potential readers of the journal, spell it out in full (in the text or a footnote) the first time it is used, with the acronym in brackets. When you're defining jargon terms or spelling out acronyms, it is normally best to do this in the text. Occasionally an expanded explanation is required that would break up the flow of the text. Many journals will not accept footnotes for such added material, but will allow a limited number of endnotes (i.e. notes at the end of the paper). Check journal policy.

A useful strategy to determine whether your argument makes sense is to write a summary sentence for each paragraph and read these sentences in sequence. In this way you can make sure that your paper has a logical flow that matches (or even improves on) your initial writing plan. Check that you have emphasised what is new or special about the contribution this paper makes to the field. In other words, sell your 'take-home' message.

Editing and revising

Editing your work is always a challenge. It is easy to see the mistakes in the work of others but difficult to find them in your own. The tendency is to read what you think is there rather than what *is* there. Reading it aloud slowly often shows up grammar and logic errors. Check your spelling and grammar. Often your computer will provide spelling and grammatical suggestions and alert you to errors. Be careful, though, to set the spell-checker to the language of the journal. English spelling differs between the UK, USA, and Australia, for example. Reduce all long sentences.

Ask friends or colleagues to read your paper for you and give you feedback. Ask them to highlight any confusing sentences and indicate where more explanation or linking is needed. Listen to what they say without becoming defensive. Revise your work so that it becomes clearer.

Preparation for submission

By now you should be satisfied with your paper but there is still quite a bit of work to be done before it is ready to send to the journal. Review the journal's information for contributors. Check carefully that you meet all the criteria (length, form of presentation, style, number of copies), and that the references are presented in the required format. Make sure you have drafted your letter appropriately (or attached the required form), addressing the journal's requirements about ownership or copyright. If you have used figures or other material that is copyrighted by another person, you need to write to them for permission to use their material, and include their response in your submission. Increasingly, journals from the health and social sciences are asking for proof of ethical clearance with articles reporting research on human subjects or animals. You must have obtained the clearance from the relevant committee *before* undertaking research. Ensure that you have made the right number of copies of the submitted manuscript and that you have all your pages properly linked if you are submitting the manuscript by email or online. This may mean that you have to scan in copies of your letter and permissions to send with your paper.

Responding to reviewers

Peer-reviewed journals send papers out to at least two reviewers for comments on its suitability for being published in the journal. This process is usually 'blind': the reviewers are not given identifying information about you, so that they can judge the paper on its merits. You will also not know the identity of the reviewers. A good reviewer reads the paper with the intention of helping you to improve it. Try not to be defensive or upset that they have criticised your work. Some of the changes they suggest may be editorial and will enhance your paper. Others might relate to content; read these carefully and follow the advice given unless the changes are inconsistent with your data or arguments.

You may discover that one reviewer likes one aspect of your paper but wants changes made to another section, while another reviewer wants changes made to the section reviewed favourably by the first reviewer. Sometimes reviewers can make inappropriate suggestions, such as asking why you did not also interview people with a similar condition to make comparisons, or advising that a different tool or method might be better. If this occurs do not panic. Write a carefully worded letter to the editor, explaining why you have chosen not to address that issue, or insert a sentence in the paper that explains more clearly why your study is limited in a particular way. Editors recognise the vagaries of the review process and will understand if you give a well-justified reason for not adopting all the suggestions of the reviewers.

Conclusion

Writing for publication can be difficult. It is challenging to get your ideas down on paper and to receive feedback on your work. Remember that your first paper may well be the hardest to write and get published, as you are learning many new skills in the process. Nevertheless, writing can be very stimulating and rewarding as you craft your ideas into a cohesive and well-substantiated argument and then see your name in print.

References

Fink, A. 2002, *How to Report on Surveys*, 2nd edn, Sage Publications, Thousand Oaks, California.

Greenwood, J. 1998, 'The "write advice" or "how to get a journal published"', *Contemporary Nurse*, vol. 7, no. 2, pp. 84–90.

Llewellyn, G. 1996, 'Reporting qualitative research', *Australian Occupational Therapy Journal*, vol. 43, pp. 178–84.

Peat, J., Elliott, E., Baur, L. & Keenan, V. 2002, *Scientific Writing: Easy When You Know How*, BMJ Books, Sydney.

Pirkis, J. & Gardner, H. 1998, 'Writing for publication', *Australian Journal of Primary Health—Interchange*, vol. 4, no. 2, pp. 71–6.

Sandler, M. P. 2003, 'The art of publishing methods', *The Journal of Nuclear Medicine*, vol. 44, no. 5, pp. 661–2.

Smith, D. 1998, 'Language and style in phenomenological research', in *Writing Qualitative Research*, ed. J. Higgs, Hampden Press, Sydney, pp. 189–95.

Watts, J. & Jackson, T. 1998, 'A task-weighted approach to determining authorship', *Australian Journal of Primary Health—Interchange*, vol. 4, no. 2, pp. 64–70.

KEY TOPICS

→ What is a thesis?

→ What makes a
good thesis?

→ How to craft and
structure a thesis

→ Matching the
writing style and
framework to the
context, genre,
and paradigm

→ Technical aspects
of writing: grammar,
language, voice,
spelling, presentation,
and layout, including
graphics and spacing

→ The writing task

Introduction

Undergraduate and postgraduate students may be involved in writing research theses (or dissertations). These are major written works. Most commonly theses are research reports but they are occasionally extensive literature reviews or a collection of the author's published research papers. Theses play a vital role in disseminating research findings. They require a special approach to scholarly writing, considering such factors as context, genre, audience, and research paradigm.

What makes a good thesis?

The term 'thesis' actually refers to the argument presented in the report and substantiated by the research. A well-written thesis therefore is an argument that is articulated clearly, based on appropriate, well-conducted research, well substantiated by the data collected, and derived logically from a sound process of data analysis and knowledge generation. The thesis should have a structure appropriate to the university and discipline in which you are studying (see below). What makes a good thesis varies also according to the degree level for which it is prepared. At undergraduate honours level, the purpose of the program is generally for students to learn about and experience well-conducted research. Part of this learning process is to develop research writing skills in writing up the thesis. At masters level a greater degree of independence is expected of students, while at doctoral level students are expected to contribute to the knowledge in their field and to conduct a substantial review of the relevant literature. Some students enrol in professional doctorate programs comprising coursework and research, programs that are commonly more practice-oriented than the PhD program.

These expectations need to be reflected in the quality and style of the thesis. Like expectations of content, expectations of the length of a thesis vary too. Table 9.1 provides a guide. (Please note that you should check these figures with your department.)

Table 9.1   Length of theses (guidelines only)

Level	Words (minimum–maximum)
Undergraduate honours	12,000–15,000, or publishable paper
Research masters	40,000–60,000
Professional doctorate	30,000–60,000
PhD	50,000–100,000

A key feature that examiners look for in every thesis is *internal consistency*: do the research questions match the paradigm, discipline genre and expectations, research methods, style of writing, and format and product of the thesis? For example, an experimental study conducted in a department of physiology would be conducted in a different style from an ethnographic study in a school of occupational therapy or an action research project in a school of nursing.

Table 9.2 summarises briefly different research paradigms, or frameworks for research. Refer to the 'Further reading' section at the end of this chapter for more information on research paradigms and approaches.

You may find it helpful to read some of the high-quality theses produced by past students in your department. Look at the style, the norms and expectations, the length, and the format. Find out if there are any particular rules you have to follow, regarding, for example, use of the first or third person in writing, the type of referencing, headings, length, format, and layout. Your supervisor or your student association could help you here (e.g. www.usyd.edu.au/supra/thesis.html). Other bodies, such as the NHMRC (National Health and Medical Research Council), provide guidelines for health and social sciences research, particularly in matters of research ethics: http://www.nhmrc.gov.au/research/general/nhmrcavc.htm.

This chapter deals with writing a thesis rather than conducting research. However, you should make sure that you read relevant books and articles about research methodology to

Table 9.2   Research paradigms

Research paradigm	Key research goals	Research approach(es)— examples	Research methods— data-collection examples	Research methods— data analysis
Empirico-analytical paradigm	To test hypotheses, identify cause–effect relationships	Experimental method, randomised controlled trials	Controlled trials, interviews, questionnaires	Statistical analysis
Interpretive paradigm	To understand, interpret, seek meaning	Phenomenology, narrative inquiry, naturalistic inquiry, arts-based inquiry	Interviews, case studies, storytelling, cognitive maps	Repeated return to data, extraction of themes, theorisation
Critical paradigm	To improve, empower, change reality or situation	Action research, collaborative research, feminist research, participatory research	Interviews, case studies, critical debate	Reflection upon data collected, action and outcomes, scholarly analysis, review by stakeholders

Source: Based on Higgs 2001

learn how best to conduct your research and to justify your research strategy when writing about it. See the 'Further reading' section at the end of this chapter for more information on research design and methodology.

How to craft and structure a thesis

In a way, creating a thesis is like writing a non-fiction story: the argument is built over an extended work involving several (often five to ten) chapters. Unlike with a story, however, you are not seeking to create suspense. Instead, you are presenting a clear, credible argument that is substantiated by sound evidence and data-analysis procedures. Structure your thesis so that your argument flows and the sections are presented in a logical manner. In the first chapter you should inform your reader what will be covered in the other chapters. This is part of creating a structure for the thesis. Remember, too, that your thesis is likely to be read in parts, because it is a long document, so you should outline briefly the purpose of each chapter at its beginning and explain how it builds on previous chapters. You may also need to provide cross-references to other parts of the thesis; for example, 'This section details the data-analysis procedures that were outlined in Section 2.3.'

Crafting the argument takes a considerable amount of work. You need to examine the literature and create a discussion that is structured in readable sections, while building up the argument in a coherent manner. Link the points within your sentences, paragraphs, and chapters clearly so that the argument within and between the chapters flows logically. If there are data, information, explanations, and definitions that the reader needs in order to understand your argument, include them in the text. By comparison, information such as ethics letters and extensive data sets is best placed in appendices (with references made to them in the main body of the thesis), so that the flow of your argument isn't disrupted (Similarly, don't use a lot of lists in the text. They break up the flow and make the reader search for the point you are trying to make.)

When structuring the thesis and building your argument, think of your thesis as both a skeleton (a set of headings that follow each other in meaningful sequence) and an extensive body of text or argument organised under these headings. Rosenthal (2002) advised that in writing a thesis you need to do the following things:

1   Introduce the thesis: tell the reader about your research and why this topic/question is of significance. Where does your study fit in the world of knowledge, particularly in your field of study?
2   Describe what you did, in sufficient detail to allow others to judge the appropriateness of your method and whether it justifies your findings.
3   Describe what you found.
4   Analyse what you found.
5   Produce a conclusion, summary, model, or set of themes that answers your research question.
6   Critically evaluate your research strategy and findings.
7   Relate your findings to the knowledge context in which your study belongs.

Not all of the above are necessarily separate sections. Table 9.3 illustrates the typical thesis structure, and some alternative headings that may be more applicable to qualitative research studies.

Table 9.3 Thesis structure

Typical thesis headings	Alternative headings for some qualitative research studies
Front pages*	Front pages*
Abstract	Abstract
Introduction	Introduction
Literature Review	Theoretical Framework
Research Methods:**	Research Strategy**
(a) Study 1	Research Findings and Discussion I (e.g. the participants' stories)
(b) Study 2 (etc.)***	Research Findings and Discussion II (e.g. a model or theory)
Results	Conclusion
Discussion	References
Conclusion	Appendices

*   These include the title page, statement of authorship (usually), acknowledgments (optional), list of figures, list of tables, glossary (optional), and table of contents (including list of appendices).

**   This includes the aims of the studies and ethics procedures.

*** Postgraduate theses may include several studies, which are commonly reported in full, in sequence.

Matching the research and writing style to the audience, genre, and paradigm

When communicating the results of your research, you should match your writing style to the context of the work. To define this context, answer the following questions: Who are the examiners likely to be (in person or in general, e.g. experts in your field of study)? Who else will read your thesis (e.g. scientists, practitioners)? What will all these people expect of it?

First, your thesis must pass the scrutiny of your *examiners*. They will judge your work, including the credibility of your research and the scholarship of your writing. Next, there are countless others who may read your thesis or publications arising from it. Consider the needs of this potential audience and how best to communicate to them.

Next, consider what style or genre is typical of your discipline (e.g. physiology, nursing, medicine). What are the expectations of the writing style of the research paradigm you have chosen? For example, experimental research is commonly written in the third person, with the actions of the researcher reported in the passive voice, and using the headings shown in the first column of Table 9.3. Qualitative research takes many forms. In some situations a particular style of writing is expected from researchers. For instance, the writing of

Table 9.4 Layout and presentation of theses

Aspect of presentation	Guidelines
Layout—paragraphs	• Use 1.5 spacing of lines (may need to be double spaced).
	• Use left justification or double justification.
	• Leave one blank line between paragraphs.
Layout—pages	• Use clear, scholarly presentation.
	• Use A4 page size.
	• Print on one side of paper only.
	• Use 2.5 cm margins, except left margin—3 cm for binding.
	• Avoid 'widows' and 'orphans' (a single or a few lines of text at the top or bottom of a page).
Binding	• You may often use soft ('perfect') binding for the examination copy.
	• Use hard (cloth) binding for the final copy.
	• Use acid-free paper for the final copy.
	• Use locally required lettering for thesis spine.
Tables and figures, appendices	• Number as per chapter (e.g. Table 3.1, Figure 3.1).
	• Tables and figures smaller than half a page may be on a page with text (don't extend them over 2 pages).
	• Place tables and figures larger than half a page on a page with no text.
	• Give clear, meaningful titles to tables, figures, and appendices.
	• All figures and tables must be mentioned in the text.
Footnotes	• Use footnotes sparingly (e.g. for definition of jargon terms and abbreviations).

phenomenologists usually demonstrates 'thick description'. In all research styles, writing should be scholarly. Watson (1987, p. 67) described the importance of such writing: 'Writing begins in freedom and ends in discipline: the self-discipline of a style.'

Technical aspects of theses

Refer to Chapter 4 (Learning Academic Writing) to refresh your mind about what is expected of your writing in terms of grammar, language, presentation, and style. When writing your thesis remember that you have a great deal resting on this one piece of assessment. You need to impress your examiners with your research, but the quality of the research can be tarnished significantly by poor technical presentation and writing. Spelling mistakes, poor grammar (especially incomplete sentences), inconsistencies, poor layout or positioning of tables and graphics, and other technical errors are not acceptable. Referencing must be meticulous.

In light of the importance of these technical aspects of presentation, it is helpful to be aware that theses generally have particular layout requirements, such as wide margins for binding. Common guidelines on presentation and layout are listed in Table 9.4, and suggested heading formats are shown in Table 9.5. Check your local rules. You should also refer to Chapter 17 (Preparing Graphics and Tables) for advice.

Table 9.5 Proposed headings for thesis

Level	Format	Font	Spacing
HEADING 1	**CHAPTER ONE or INTRODUCTION**	Capitals, bold, larger e.g. 18 point	Centred, space below
HEADING 2	**1.1 SECTION ONE**	Capitals, bold	LHS, space above
HEADING 3	**1.1.1 Sub-Section One**	Title case,* bold	LHS
HEADING 4	**A) Subheading**	Sentence case,** bold	LHS
HEADING 5	1) Subheading next	Sentence case,** italics	LHS

LHS = Left-hand-side justified.

*   *Title case* means that all the words apart from 'the', 'a', 'of', 'and', etc., are capitalised.

** *Sentence case* headings start with a capital letter, but all the subsequent words (apart from Proper Nouns) are lowercase.

The writing task

The task of writing includes four phases: preparation, writing, reflection/critique, and proofing/printing.

Preparation

In the preparation phase you need to do the following things:
*   Investigate your topic.
*   Keep track of the information and literature you collect.
*   Choose a good referencing strategy (computer files are preferable).
*   Choose a referencing system (e.g. Harvard, Vancouver, or your university's style).
*   Keep meticulous records of your references.

- Conduct your research.
- Develop a style guide.
- Organise access to good computer hardware and software: you don't want to have to re-type text or spend a lot of time translating files into new software systems.
- Set up a 'custom dictionary' in your word processing software; as you save your work, add key words to your dictionary to avoid having to check words or names you use frequently each time you spell-check.

Writing

In the writing phase you need to do the following:
- Plan your argument.
- Organise your literature and data into a sequence/structure for writing.
- Develop a plan for writing.
- Create one file per chapter. Avoid large files, because you will lose a lot of work and time if they become corrupted.
- Back up electronic files regularly and store back-up copies in more than one place for safety.

Writing a major work can be daunting and you may experience writer's block. Watson (1987, pp. 38–9) gave the following advice on dealing with writer's block: 'The first step is to recall that writing is not a single process and not a single act, and that there is no reasonable presumption that any single sentence should come right in its first draft. ... The life of an author is mostly a matter of pushing the words about on the page—altering, re-ordering, adding, deleting, refining.'

Strategies that you can use to help with your writing (particularly with a large and complex document like a thesis) include the following:
- Brainstorm (i.e. collect all your ideas on the topic).
- Develop a flowchart or concept map to organise your thoughts.
- Write up a draft table of contents and write under these headings.
- Write down your broad ideas on the topic and progressively refine them, to develop an argument, and then structure the information logically to support and present this argument.
- Write in 'bite-sized' sections.
- Just write! Don't worry if it's not good enough the first time. Once you start writing, you will have something to refine and polish later.

Writing the literature review poses some particular challenges. Burnard (1992, p. 101) offered these suggestions:

> When you write up your research review, try to avoid the rather dull listing of everything you have read. The aim of a literature review is not only to identify what you have read, but for you to offer a critical review of what you have read. ... comment on the findings that you report. Offer a critique (of the research method) ... Indicate in what ways [other] researchers' findings fit in with your study.

Reflection/critique

In the reflection/critique phase it is good to do the following:
- Put your writing aside for a while so that you can look at it again with a fresh, critical mind.
- Read your work aloud so that you can see where it doesn't make sense, where more clarity is needed, and where you have made grammatical errors (such as incomplete sentences).
- Ask someone else (a 'critical friend') to read your work and give you feedback.
- Check that your thesis is well argued, grounded in data, and well referenced.

Proofing/printing

In the proofing/printing phase you should carry out the following tasks:

- Proofread your work. Spell-check it (but remember that the computer cannot tell you if you have confused words such as 'were' and 'where').
- Format your work consistently.
- Decide which printer, computer, and software you will use to print your final copy. Remember that different printers paginate differently and if you plan your layout for one printer and then print on another your page breaks may not coincide with the new printer layout and you could be left with a few lines only at the top of a page.
- Paginate your work, ensuring that figures and tables are placed appropriately and pages are numbered sequentially, and checking that the page numbers of pages set out in 'landscape' format are positioned appropriately.
- Check the print-out as it is being printed for layout and page numbering.

For more on how to write a research thesis, refer to the 'Further reading' section at the end of this chapter.

Making the most of your supervisor

Your supervisor has five key roles in relation to your research program. He or she:

- knows how the administrative system works, and can help with such tasks as enrolment, meeting the deadlines and requirements of the program, keeping on target with specific tasks, getting ethics approval, finding appropriate examiners, and preparing your thesis for examination
- helps you get access to research infrastructure (including resources, funding, scholarships, and resource people)
- has knowledge in your topic area and/or knows people who can help you learn more about your topic
- knows how to do research and is a guide and role model for you
- provides feedback on your work: on your research design and activities, your findings and how you are interpreting them, and your writing.

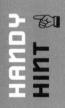

9.1 Working with your research supervisor

- Remember your supervisor is there to help you; ask for help whenever you need it.
- Take an agenda or a list of questions to your meetings with your supervisor. It helps to be organised.
- Negotiate dates with your supervisor for handing in your writing and getting feedback about your work.
- Ask your supervisor for help or advice about accessing resources, funding, and resource people. Your supervisor knows how the system works.

HANDY HINT

Where to from here?

Research can be rewarding and also challenging. Spend some time thinking about your tasks and the people who can help you. Learn to balance learning about research (reading, attending training sessions, etc.) with getting on with it. You want to complete your work in a timely fashion, rather than be overloaded with tasks like 'writing up' or data processing as you rapidly approach your submission deadline. Writing a thesis is a major task in itself, alongside and as part of your research. It needs planning, structuring, and rigour as well as style.

References

Burnard, P. 1992, *Writing for Health Professionals: A Manual for Writers*, Chapman & Hall, London.
Higgs, J. 2001, 'Charting standpoints in qualitative research', in *Critical Moments in Qualitative Research*, eds H. Byrne-Armstrong, J. Higgs & D. Horsfall, Butterworth-Heinemann, Oxford, pp. 44–67.
Rosenthal, J. 2002, 'Notes on academic writing: Writing with style', course notes for graduate students, School of Physiotherapy, The University of Sydney.
Watson, G. 1987, *Writing a Thesis: A Guide to Long Essays and Dissertations*, Longman, London.

Further reading

Research paradigms and approaches

Denzin, N. K. & Lincoln, Y. S. 2000, 'Introduction: The discipline and practice of qualitative research', in *Handbook of Qualitative Research*, 2nd edn, eds N. K. Denzin & Y. S. Lincoln, Sage Publications, London, pp. 1–28.
Lincoln, Y. S. & Guba, E. G. 2000, 'Paradigmatic controversies, contradictions, and emerging confluences', in *Handbook of Qualitative Research*, 2nd edn, eds N. K. Denzin & Y. S. Lincoln, Sage Publications, London, pp. 163–88.
Minichiello, V., Sullivan, G., Greenwood, K. & Axford, R. (eds) 2003, *Handbook of Research Methods in Health Sciences*, Addison-Wesley, Sydney.

Research design and methodology

Balnaves, M. & Caputi, P. 2001, *Introduction to Quantitative Research Methods: An Investigative Approach*, Sage Publications, London.
Booth, W., Colomb, G. G. & Williams, J. M. 2003, *Craft of Research*, 2nd edn, University of Chicago Press, Chicago.
Denzin, N. K. & Lincoln, Y. S. (eds) 2000, *Handbook of Qualitative Research*, 2nd edn, Sage Publications, Thousand Oaks, California.
Ezzy, D. 2002, *Qualitative Analysis: Practice and Innovation*, Allen and Unwin, Crows Nest, NSW.
Flick, U. 2002, *An Introduction to Qualitative Research*, 2nd edn, Sage Publications, London.
Gillham, B. 2000, *The Research Interview*, Continuum, London.
Hammell, K. W., Carpenter, C. & Dyck, I. (eds) 2000, *Using Qualitative Research: A Practical Introduction for Occupational and Physical Therapists*, Churchill Livingstone, London.
Huck, S. W. 2000, *Reading Statistics and Research*, 3rd edn, Longman, New York.
McNiff, S. 2000, *Art-based Research*, Jessica Kingsley Publishers, London.
Polgar, S. & Thomas, S. A. 2000, *Introduction to Research in the Health Sciences*, 4th edn, Churchill Livingstone, Edinburgh.
Thomas, R. M. 2003, *Blending Qualitative and Quantitative Research Methods in Theses and Dissertations*, Corwin Press, Thousand Oaks, California.

Writing a research thesis

Burnard, P. 1992, *Writing for Health Professionals: A Manual for Writers*, Chapman & Hall, London.
Glatthorn, A. A. 1998, *Writing the Winning Dissertation: A Step-by-Step Guide*, Corwin Press, London.
Holliday, A. 2002, *Doing and Writing Qualitative Research*, Sage Publications, London.
Preece, R. A. 1994, *Starting Research: An Introduction to Academic Research and Dissertation Writing*, Pinter Publishers, London.

Wallace, A., Schirato, T. & Bright, P. 1999, *Beginning University: Thinking, Researching and Writing for Success*, Allen & Unwin, St Leonards, NSW.

Wolfe, J. 1996, *How to Write a PhD Thesis*, © University of New South Wales, <http:/www.phys. unsw.edu.au/~jw/thesis.html> accessed 24 August 2003.

10 ELECTRONIC COMMUNICATION AND COMMUNICATING IN FLEXIBLE LEARNING

Mary Jane Mahony

KEY TOPICS

→ Understanding flexible learning environments and resources

→ Planning for flexible learning

→ Learning to communicate in flexible learning

Introduction

Studying in the health and social sciences is very likely to involve you in new methods of communication because of:

- the wide range of learning resources available in higher education
- opportunities for interacting with professional practitioners and other industry experts who are located off-campus
- professional practice placements away from campus
- the demands of managing your studies along with other responsibilities (work, family, community, sport)
- expectations that as a graduate you will be prepared for involvement in tele-practice and tele-education activities.

This chapter deals with two key aspects of flexible learning: communication and flexible learning environments. 'Flexible' refers to flexibility in mode, time, place, etc.: 'distance', 'electronic', 'multi-mode', 'distributed', 'online', 'blended', or 'off campus' learning and communication. The common characteristic of flexible learning programs is that you won't be learning in the traditional classroom with a traditional timetable and you will be using a range of communication methods. This will mirror some of your likely communication experiences as a professional. While telemedicine has led the way in using all forms of electronic conferencing (e.g. consultations with specialists remote from the general practitioner and/or client's location), the use of electronic communication is becoming ubiquitous for busy people, particularly professional practitioners, who may also be geographically dispersed or simply working on different shifts.

As a student in a flexible learning program you may be communicating with other students and your teachers from home, your workplace, a library or computer access centre, or some other location. You are often likely to be using some form of information/communication technology and you are likely to be on your own. Your fellow students and your teachers (and perhaps other expert contributors) will usually be at a distance in location and time, although sometimes you might meet with other students in block/intensive-mode on-campus classes. You will need to be self-disciplined and to practise adept time management and priority setting.

In this chapter I emphasise the importance of taking control and being responsible for your part in making these communications and learning activities effective. I introduce you to some forms of communication (asynchronous and synchronous) and what they may require of you. I also include some tips on how to use these modes efficiently and effectively.

Taking control: planning and organising for success

Flexible learning differs from traditional classroom delivery and timetabling, where it is easy to follow what others are doing. In the traditional situation you normally attend class once a week, at a specified time, and the expectations for each class are set out. Flexible learning, on the other hand, is usually much less organised. It does not impose a fixed timetable and place for learning. You need to decide these things for yourself, including when you will participate in class discussions.

10.1   Planning and organising your studies

- Construct a weekly study timetable for yourself that includes all activities, including learning how to use new technology. (Refer to Chapter 2 for detailed advice on how to draw up a study timetable.)
- Acknowledge that you need to allocate regular periods of time to your studies. Flexible learning gives you more control but does not reduce the time and effort needed.
- Ask for help early (regardless of whether you think it may be a 'dumb question').

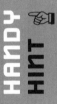

HANDY HINT

Finding your way through your learning resources

You are likely to need and be asked to cope with a range of resources for learning. Figure 10.1 illustrates some of the possibilities. Some may be 'packaged' resources (e.g. books, collected readings, videos, and kits) to be used in your learning as directed. Others will be opportunities for interactive communication (e.g. telephone tutorials, email, and Web-supported discussion forums).

Figure 10.1 What your flexible learning environment may include

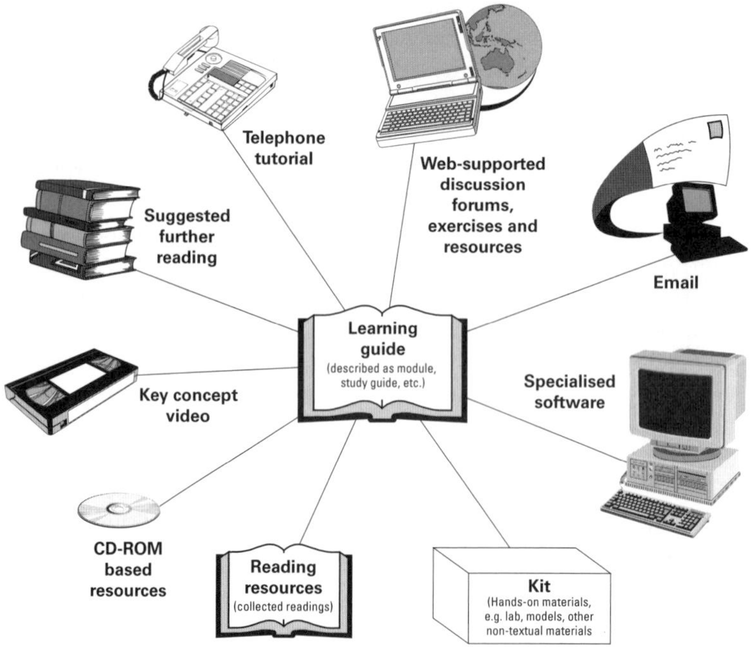

Note: This diagram was prepared using Inspiration®, a useful software tool for organising and communicating
ideas. See www.inspiration.com (accessed 5 April 2004).

Your first responsibility is to be clear about what is expected of you. Your core directions usually appear in a learning guide (this appears centrally in Figure 10.1), provided
either on paper or electronically. Due dates for assignments are easy to put in your diary.
Determining when and what other learning activities are necessary and putting them in
your diary may require careful consideration of all the learning resources available to you.

You already use print on paper in many ways. The advice in this chapter includes advice
on using print appropriately in academic situations where electronic media are used. (You'll
find advice about using written text in specific academic forms of communication in other
chapters in this book.)

The online/multimedia environment

'Going online' usually means going on the Web. You will certainly use multimedia on the
Web, which includes a mixture of media, such as text, animation, video, and audio. You may
also work offline. CD-ROMs and DVDs are often used for convenience or to save the time
and costs involved in downloading information and long files (such as video sequences), particularly via modem. Whether you are studying online or offline, you may find that many
pathways and sequences become possible and some new skills are needed. Even if you are
an experienced Web surfer, you may be less sure about what happens when you enter a
'structured learning environment', sometimes known as a learning management system.
(Educational institutions may use proprietary systems such as WebCT or BlackBoard, or
may have constructed their own. You will usually enter by logging on with your student ID

and password.) Online activities may require you to acknowledge some skill deficits (and even a lack of confidence). Tackling these up-front will reduce your stress level and probably eliminate one source of procrastination and frustration.

Explore the CD-ROM or website for your course and check out the information and tools available. These are neither books nor classrooms, though they may offer elements of both. Be prepared to play around until you feel comfortable; don't be scared of making mistakes. Become comfortable with the Web browser you use, and become familiar with the technical support it offers. For example, you can mark a Web address so you can return to it easily, place links to frequently visited websites on a visible toolbar, and open multiple windows so that you have easy access to several Web pages at the same time.

Ask for advice and clarification if you need it. Try to distinguish between technical and academic matters. Technical assistance for accessing and working in the online environment is usually available from help desks or local technical staff. Academic matters relate to the content of your studies or to packaged resources such as readings, videos, and CD-ROMs; questions about these matters are best addressed to teaching staff. Of course, you can also ask a friend, spouse, or child who has more experience in these areas than you. Then, organise your studies in a timetable that suits you, and get ready to communicate!

Asynchronous communication or learning mode

In flexible learning you will still interact with your teachers and fellow learners, in tutorials, group discussions, presentations, and collaborative project work. Most commonly, you'll be expected to use email and/or Web-based discussion groups; occasionally you may use voicemail. These are tools for communication among people separated by time, space, or both. Asynchronous means 'not at the same time'. Asynchronous communication gives you the opportunity to think about what others have said and what you want to say, without the pressure to contribute immediately before the discussion moves on. In planning your schedule, first consider your own needs and availability, then consider how you can complete tasks

Table 10.1   Comparing asynchronous and synchronous communication

Asynchronous communication	
Advantages	**Disadvantages**
• You have a record of the communication (yours and others).	• You may have to pay connection costs (Internet service provider, telephone connection, etc.) or travel to the computer.
• You choose a time that suits you (within a general timetable) and manage any scheduling conflicts.	• You may have to upgrade your computer system so that it meets the technical specifications for the online learning program and delivers efficient and trouble-free communication.
• You have time to reflect on what you read and what you write.	
• You choose the place (depending on your access to a suitably equipped computer).	• You may need to develop your computer skills.
• You develop your computer skills and confidence.	• You may feel frustration if your keyboard skills are slow.
	• You may become frustrated waiting for others to contribute or dissatisfied with their level of contribution.

Table 10.1 Comparing asynchronous and synchronous communication (continued)

Synchronous communication	
Advantages	**Disadvantages**
• You have the opportunity to interact immediately with your fellow students and your teachers, and to receive immediate feedback on your communication.	• You must adhere to a set schedule.
	• You may have connection costs or travel costs. These depend on the communication media used.
• You choose the place (depending on the technology used).	• You may have to upgrade your computer system so that it meets the technical specifications for the online learning program and delivers fast, efficient, and trouble-free communication.
• You may have a record of the event. Use of audio, or audio with video, may enhance your social experience with fellow students and your teachers.	
	• In chat and instant messaging, you may feel frustrated or left behind if your keyboard skills are slow or if others take over the discussion.
	• In audio- or video-conferencing (especially desktop), you may find the standard of picture or sound unsatisfactory for the intended communication.

(such as reading others' contributions and posting your input to weekly online discussions) that are important to other students and the teacher as well as you. Table 10.1 compares asynchronous communication with synchronous communication by showing the advantages and disadvantages of each.

Always remember to ACT: *Ask* if things are unclear; *Contribute* ideas, constructive comment, and information you have found useful; and *Think* about what other people have posted. Take pride in what you post. Think about what is required to be an effective message sender and receiver.

HANDY HINT ☞

10.2 Sending electronic messages

- Compose the 'subject' to give the essence of your message and assist in retrieval. An ideal subject line provides keywords that best characterise the contents of the message and/or link the message to a previous thread.
- If you are replying and are changing the topic or direction of the discussion, use a new subject title.
- Keep your paragraphs short, to make your emails easy to read on computer screens. Paragraphs can usually be a bit more fluid in online conversations than in an essay.
- Offer reasons for your criticisms and support for your claims, and include pointers to sources of further information.
- Quote selectively; include only enough of previous messages for your reply to be understood.

- Make how you feel, as well as what you think, visible. Brief statements such as 'I laughed out loud when …' or 'I felt uncomfortable when …', or common emoticons such as the smiley face :-) or the sad face :-(can also help in informal communication. This more casual language should not be used when you are communicating with your teachers (e.g. submitting assignments or asking questions about your studies or enrolment).
- Don't use the abbreviations commonly used in online and text-messaging social inter-actions (e.g. '4U'). You are communicating in an academic or professional environment.
- Don't use all capital letters. That is considered to be like shouting.
- Avoid losing your work if your online connection times out or drops out. Compose your more thoughtful, complex, or substantial messages in a word processing document, then copy and paste them into an email message or discussion-group posting.
- If you include an attachment, give it an informative, unique name.
- Before you hit SEND, be sure your message is going only to the person/s you want to have read it. Hitting REPLY thoughtlessly has embarrassed many electronic communicators.
- Remember, you are communicating with people. Offer your online colleagues courtesy and respect. Treat others as you would wish to be treated.

10.3   Receiving electronic messages

HANDY HINT

- Acknowledge emails received. A brief 'thanks' assures the sender that you have received the message.
- Avoid replying in haste or in heat; think over your contribution before sending it. Composing your message offline helps.
- Develop time-management strategies so you do not feel overwhelmed. For example, designate specific times to check and respond to email.
- Develop file-management strategies. Learn to name electronic files and folders sys-tematically. You need to be comfortable with saving and managing files and folders. In Windows environments use Windows Explorer. Consult your computer's help menus for assistance or ask a more experienced friend to help you.
- Give senders feedback when their communication creates problems for you (e.g. it is hard to understand or the language is inappropriate).
- Acknowledge contributions of fellow students appropriately when you refer to them in formal written work, and get permission to quote them if you are using their words other than in your immediate learning.

Synchronous communication or learning mode

Communicating together in real time (via teleconferencing, face-to-face learning, online learning, etc.) is called 'synchronous communication'. Getting together online and at the same time is synchronous communication. It is immediate, without breaks to wait and see what someone will say next. In flexible learning you are most likely to experience it through participating in a chat room (synchronous text conferencing), a telephone con-ference (synchronous voice conferencing), or videoconferencing (synchronous visual and voice conferencing). Blocks (e.g. one week) of on–campus learning can also be considered synchronous, face-to-face communication and learning. Videoconferencing may be conventional (rooms are connected using specialist videoconferencing equipment), desktop (computers are outfitted with appropriate software and hardware connections), or a mixture of the two.

Desktop conferencing using, for example, MSN Messenger, Windows NetMeeting, and the Internet allows you to blend these communication facilities at your computer desktop, though they are not yet widely used for education. Although communication connections between two computers via the Internet are simple to manage, multiple-site audio and/or video communication requires special equipment and may not be technically or financially feasible. Sharing text and graphics via the Internet can be easy, but managing a voice or video connection can be a challenge.

10.4   Learning to communicate in different media

Distance/flexible communication

- When meeting to videoconference, etc., be there ahead of the scheduled time. Double-check if you are located in a different time zone, to be sure you know what local time you are due to commence.
- Read all instructions provided in advance, to increase your confidence and minimise surprises. This includes completing pre-reading, preparation for tutorial discussion, etc.
- Practise informally with others to increase your familiarity with the technological aspects of the meeting.

Voicemail

- Add the identifying data that online communication usually provides automatically: your name, the time and date of the call, specific details on the topic of your message, and your contact details.
- Spell out your name if it is difficult and repeat any phone numbers and other contact details.

Chat rooms

- If you are making a presentation, prepare it in advance, then copy and paste it into a message.
- Use short messages with a sign indicating that receivers should continue the discussion (usually a +), to minimise waiting time for other participants.

Telephone conferencing

- You may be connected individually at your own handset or speaker phone, or with a group of others at a single location and using loudspeaker equipment.
- Send any illustrations you might want to use to all participants ahead of time.
- Ensure you have a quiet background for the period of the call. Turn off the television and other noisemakers; remove dogs and small children from the discussion room.
- Arrange to sit somewhere where you can write.
- Have your pen, notepaper, and required materials for the call ready in advance.
- Turn off 'call-waiting' if you make use of such a telephone service.

- Speak distinctly during the conference and with your mouth close to the handset if you are using one. The moderator will give feedback on whether you are too loud or too soft.
- Make a conscious effort to put 'colour' into your voice; let your voice indicate when you are smiling.
- If in a group, help with communicating the group's responses; for example, 'Everyone here nodded in agreement with your views.' From time to time, ask for an indication of the nonverbals; for example, 'I wish I could see you, you sound like you are happy/puzzled. Are you?'
- Always introduce yourself when taking a turn: 'It's Mary Jane speaking.' Don't be afraid to ask who is speaking if they do not introduce themselves. It helps you situate the content and tone of interaction.

Conventional videoconferencing

- Normally, you will participate in a videoconference at a managed location. Staff there will advise you.
- Be confident. Sit close to camera, microphones, and screen: you'll feel more a part of the action than if you are at the back of the room.
- Have appropriately prepared illustrations and overheads if you are to present. Ask for guidance ahead of time if instructions are not provided.
- Identify yourself and address participants at other locations by name.

Desktop conferencing

- You are likely to be personally in charge of the technology at your site, unless it is in a purpose-specific site, such as a hospital, clinic, or other institution. You should be told what computer resources you will need for a successful conference and what procedures you must follow to be connected. Be sure to prepare in advance. All the tips above are relevant.
- Practise ahead of time to ensure you are comfortable with the basic procedures and their implications. For example, ensure you are familiar with the process for displaying files on your computer to other participants during the conference. Will people understand it? Would a diagram help?
- If you are presenting, ensure that your document (whether in a presentation, word processing, spreadsheet, or other application) is not overloaded with graphics, which may prevent other participants from viewing it easily.

Be careful with email

The use of email for professional communication can create problems in meeting expectations about politeness. We probably have all had the experience of receiving an email from a friend or colleague and wondering if we have upset them in some way, because the email is short and sharp. Emails allow for, and in fact encourage, brief and informal communication. When time pressure exaggerates this trend to brevity, the result can be disconcerting for the reader. When emailing to someone from another country or culture, take care to write in an appropriate style in terms of the degree of politeness and formality (e.g. use of first names). It can be helpful to consult a guide on 'netiquette' for the rules of good cyberspace communication.

Conclusion

Communicating in flexible learning environments, using some form of information or communication technology, may be challenging at first, but the benefits are many. You will usually be able to interact (socially and academically) with everyone in your learning environment, at times and places that suit you, including people you might not otherwise have the opportunity of meeting.

There have been some recurring themes in the advice given this chapter:

- Plan and prepare in advance.
- Ask for help early.
- Practise ahead of time with any technology that is new to you.
- Make *your* contribution.

Your experiences communicating in these ways will prepare you for the increasingly wired world of health and social science professionals.

Further reading

Tyler, S., Kossen, C. & Ryan, C. 2002, *Communication: A Foundation Course*, 2nd edn, Prentice Hall Australia, Sydney.

'Using the Internet: Netiquette' <http://www.sofweb.vic.edu.au/internet/netiquet.htm> accessed 22 March 2004.

'Welcome to the web' <http://www.teachingideas.co.uk/welcome/> accessed 5 April 2004.

Windschuttle, K. & Elliott, E.1999, *Writing, Researching and Communicating: Communication Skills for the Information Age*, 3rd edn, McGraw-Hill, Sydney.

COMMUNICATING in PROBLEM-BASED LEARNING CLASSES

Ann Sefton

KEY TOPICS

→ Problem-based learning (PBL) as an active, self-directed learning process

→ The roles of students and tutors in PBL

→ Effective and supportive behaviour in PBL tutorials

→ Giving and receiving appropriate feedback on the processes

Introduction

Problem-based learning (PBL) is increasingly being implemented in health and social sciences curricula. This chapter focuses on clinical problem solving in PBL programs; the general strategies are applicable to other PBL classes in professional-education courses. Students are active participants in these programs, constructing their own understanding and determining their learning agendas. To be effective, the process requires styles of participation, interaction, and learning different from those of traditional university classrooms. Mutual trust and support are essential. In this chapter you will learn what characterises PBL and how you can make the most of the method. Effective learning involves critical thinking, active participation and collaboration, and the capacity to take responsibility for your learning.

What is PBL?

PBL is a specific method of case-based, active learning. The process encourages understanding of underlying mechanisms in health and disease by modelling clinical problem solving. Students work cooperatively as a team, a common situation for health professionals. Since its development at McMaster University in Canada, PBL has been adopted widely.

PBL requires students to work in small groups to explore and resolve clinical problems devised by staff. Each problem typically extends for a week, sometimes longer. Tutors do not teach content knowledge, but facilitate the learning process. PBL has been shown to be effective in supporting students' self-directed learning, and in enhancing other skills: communicating, confidently using clinical and scientific language, integrating knowledge, practising critical reasoning, and identifying gaps in personal understanding. The key is that students actively direct their own learning and share with colleagues.

The richness of PBL comes from the integration of underlying scientific and clinical issues with broad social, community, and professional contexts. Also, information is shared within the group to help reach a resolution. PBL is most effective when it is integrated across disciplines (reflecting the reality of patients' problems), but occasionally variants of PBL are used within a single subject, perhaps relating to complex issues and research questions.

The role of a PBL tutor

It is important to appreciate the tutor's responsibilities in PBL. Tutors facilitate the learning process and encourage all students to participate. They should provide neither substantial didactic information nor indicate that ideas are 'right' or 'wrong', although they will subtly encourage the group to review unclear or dubious statements. When groups are working smoothly, tutors may intervene only rarely. PBL offers the potential for extensive communication between and among the members of the group; tutors ensure smooth interactions and encourage a single shared conversation. They empower quieter members and may make suggestions when the conversation stalls. Sometimes they help the group to manage an over-enthusiastic, dominant, or even disruptive personality. In a review of each problem, tutors invite the students to make comments on the group's progress, and provide feedback and make suggestions. It is important for discussion to be honest, but also for everyone to be sensitive to the feelings of others.

Your tutor might interview all group members individually in order to discuss each student's contribution, to develop knowledge, and to address concerns. Such sessions are valuable. A perceptive tutor will offer insightful comments about your progress, highlighting your strengths and weaknesses so as to enhance your skills in group settings. Occasionally, in some environments, each student's performance in tutorials is graded. This is unusual in PBL as it may inhibit the free exchange of information. If you are subject to such assessments, be sure that you understand the expectations very clearly and don't let it inhibit your participation.

The PBL process

The PBL cycle begins when the student group is introduced to the problem. In health and social sciences, the problem, usually developed around a patient, may emphasise diagnosis, management, or social issues, depending on the focus of the profession. Groups typically meet two or three times for discussion. The tutor may reveal information progressively in tutorials, or further data may be presented on paper or via the Web, particularly if tutorial time is limited. In some programs, an online discussion board (e.g. WebCT or BlackBoard) is used to facilitate the learning process, particularly if people are out in the field and want to link back into the support network.

A 'trigger' is presented on paper, film, video, or computer, perhaps supported by images. Triggers may be short (like the one below), stimulating immediate interaction and responses. Alternatively, substantial and detailed information may be provided in an initial handout of a page or so, to which the students react systematically, identifying learning issues. Either way, the result is usually lively discussion, the generation of hypotheses, and the identification of areas of ignorance or confusion.

An example of a short trigger

CASE STUDY 11.1

Antonio Rinaldo, aged 8, presents in distress at the local dentist's surgery with his mother after falling off his skateboard in the park an hour ago. His mouth is bleeding and his mother has one of his teeth in a handkerchief.

Brainstorming, a typical group would raise the following issues: How do we deal with his distress? What are the first things we should say to him and his mother? Where is the bleeding coming from? Is it a 'baby tooth'? What should we do with the tooth? Is it possible to re-implant it? What about germs? He has a Mediterranean name: might that be significant? What do we need to know about his family? And so on. These issues are prioritised before the group goes on to develop a set of questions to ask Antonio and his mother.

Although in PBL the discussion is free-flowing and lively, there is an underlying structure to it. One example model or structure for a diagnostic problem is illustrated in Figure 11.1. After the trigger, a brainstorming session ensures that issues are identified and noted, usually on a whiteboard. It is important initially to think broadly and record the ideas. Those listed are subsequently organised and scrutinised critically in a general discussion. The group rejects obviously incorrect or unlikely possibilities. Hypotheses are then generated to try to explain the key data presented in the trigger. During these processes, the group identifies and records learning issues that members will need to understand to advance toward resolution of the problem. As a group member, you may note additional items for your individual follow-up after the class meetings.

When the group breaks up, students study the issues identified, using textbooks or resources provided (e.g. online or in libraries) to advance their understanding. Cooperative learning groups can be very effective. Practical classes, lectures, seminars, skills sessions, or clinical encounters may be provided to help students to understand the issues raised by the problem.

The group reassembles for members to share their new understanding in discussion, and to identify and organise further information needed from the 'patient'. In response to appropriate questions, the tutor may provide information, or offer a handout or online access to data. The group agrees on a tentative diagnosis (if that is the focus) and usually considers principles of management, taking into account geographic and social factors. In discussion, the group usually identifies additional learning issues for individual study. A final resolution is agreed jointly.

Figure 11.1 Conceptual model of the PBL process

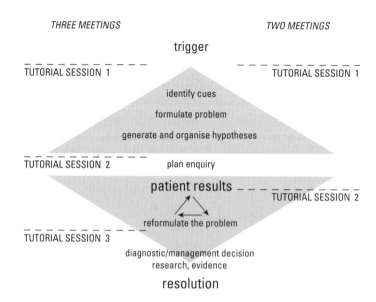

The model illustrates how the PBL process starts from a trigger and broadens out to include a wide range of issues, before narrowing to a final resolution. The model is modified from earlier diagrams from the Faculties of Medicine at the Universities of Newcastle and Sydney. It illustrates typical break points (dotted lines), depending on whether there are two or three tutorials for the problem. The arrows indicate that issues are reviewed and discussed during a process of refining the ideas generated from the history, symptoms, and signs, and the results of investigations.

Students' roles in a PBL group

You have a responsibility to contribute actively but sensitively to the problem-solving process. When a new group forms, it is a good idea to agree on some simple expectations with the tutor. While it is important to challenge ideas, the PBL process depends on mutual trust and respect for others. Everyone must have a chance to express their ideas. In groups, the collective knowledge may be enough to resolve the problem, but that understanding must be transferred to each individual.

Most groups elect a secretary to ensure that information is passed between tutor and students and to carry out tasks on behalf of the group (e.g. collecting materials and representing the group at reviews and focus discussions). Make sure the secretary has everyone's email and phone contact details. At each tutorial, a scribe records the discussion (on a whiteboard, for example) by summarising and organising the points raised, so that important ideas are not lost. It is customary to rotate this task around the group, as it develops valuable skills of critical listening, comprehension, and summarising.

When the problem 'trigger' is introduced, everyone contributes to the brainstorming, discussion, and refining of ideas. If you have particular knowledge of the subject, it can sometimes be frustrating not to take over, but everyone needs to participate and develop their own and the group's understanding.

After each tutorial, you will usually identify key issues to study. While some groups divide up the initial research, remember that all members have to acquire the essential knowledge for themselves. At the next tutorial, presenting and discussing the information is important to ensure that all members are up to speed on the key issues that you have agreed to study. You should feel comfortable questioning ideas that seem unclear or incorrect, and expanding on others when you have specific knowledge. Be sure that everyone's reasoning is clear, but remember to confine any criticisms you have to the content, not the individual presenting it. You have an obligation to participate in feedback sessions (commonly held at the end of each problem). You will usually be expected to complete evaluation forms and it is important to give honest opinions. Try, however, to suggest improvements rather than simply offer damning criticism.

11.1 Working in PBL groups

HANDY HINT

- Treat the other members of your learning group with respect and honesty; you can expect the same from them.
- Be prepared both to listen and to take your turn in discussion. While you must avoid putting your colleagues down, it is important to critique faulty logic and to challenge information you think is wrong.
- You have an obligation to work on the group's agreed study topics, not only for yourself but also to contribute to later discussion. Work out early for yourself which textbooks are most appropriate and use them. Consult any Web-based resources provided and check the validity and reliability of sites you find yourself.
- You may find it particularly helpful to work informally with a few other students in a cooperative learning group outside tutorials.
- Be prepared to reflect on the group's progress and on your own performance. Contribute to evaluation sessions each week.
- Suggest ways to improve the group's work, but be sensitive to the feelings of others. Positive suggestions are usually better received than negative remarks.
- Think carefully about any criticism of your contributions; don't just assume that it is ill-informed or wrong. Reflect on any personal feedback you receive and seek further advice from the tutor or your colleagues if you need it.
- Be prepared to (tactfully) raise issues of concern about the group's functioning, the tutor's style, or the process itself. Complete evaluation forms if asked.

Being a good group member

Your active participation is essential: the PBL process is based on sharing. Offer to share the different roles; you will find it a rewarding experience. Be careful not to dominate, even when you have special knowledge or experience. On the other hand, avoid being passive. You will learn most by actively suggesting and exploring ideas, even if they turn out to be wrong. Although some of your group may not be particular friends of yours, everyone brings something to the group. In professional life you will usually not be able to choose the members of working teams. (See Chapter 22 for a discussion of group dynamics and roles of group members.)

Attendance at PBL tutorials is usually compulsory, because of the emphasis on the group and its progress. If you have to miss a tutorial, notify the tutor; the group can keep you informed of its progress. Be prepared to offer the same support to others.

Managing your time is particularly important. It is easy to become absorbed in certain fascinating issues but you must ensure that you understand and learn the core elements of the problem. Study plans are particularly important (see Chapter 2). If you find interesting information, be sure to record it accurately so that you can find it again.

Issues in PBL

Students in PBL programs are sometimes unclear about what to learn and how much depth is required. If goals seem unclear, discuss them within your group and ask staff for clarification. Take advantage of any guidelines on skills, competencies, or the depth and breadth of knowledge. Use formative assessments (trial examinations, past papers, or questions on the Web) to identify your strengths and weaknesses without penalty. You will gain confidence by doing them.

If English is not your first language and you are not confident in oral communication, let the group know and ask them to ensure that you are included. Seek help from the relevant university resource centre as early as possible; staff there will offer support that will benefit all your studies, as well as later communication with patients and clinicians.

The presence of a disruptive member or interpersonal issues between members can create difficulties. Raise concerns frankly but sensitively, and encourage the group and the tutor to explore solutions. The group may also need to consider approaching (tactfully) a tutor who intervenes too much or too little. At worst, remember that group members (and tutors) often rotate each term or semester!

Conclusion

In many courses students participate in PBL. The method is both effective and enjoyable (see Boud & Feletti 1991). We hope you make the most of your PBL experiences.

References

Boud, D. J. & Feletti, G. (eds) 1991, *The Challenge of Problem-based Learning*, 2nd edn, Kogan Page, London.

Bullimore, D. W. 1998, 'Tutorials and small group work', in D. W. Bullimore (ed.), *Study Skills and Tomorrow's Doctors*, W. B. Saunders, Edinburgh, pp. 84–90.

Woods, D. R. 1994, *Problem-based Learning: How to Gain the Most from PBL*, D. R. Woods, Box 762, Waterdown, ON l0R 2H0, Canada.

12 | WRITING RECORDS, REPORTS, AND REFERRALS IN PROFESSIONAL PRACTICE

Lindy McAllister, Iain Hay, and Annette Street

KEY TOPICS

→ Writing professional documents: a developmental skill for all students and practitioners

→ Different genres, purposes, and types of reports, records, and referrals in the health and social science professions

→ Writing for different audiences (e.g. lecturers, fieldwork educators, patients, other health professionals, school teachers, and peers)

→ Different structures for different types of writing

→ Avoiding ethical and medico-legal problems when committing information to paper

→ Strategies for effective report writing

Introduction

One of the core skills for health and social science professionals is the ability to write reports, records, and referrals that are clear, succinct, informative, and useful, that address the practitioner's responsibility to communicate professionally and meet their duty of care, and that avoid ethical and legal pitfalls. This is a skill that develops over time, beginning in the student years and continuing to improve with practice as a professional.

In this chapter we use the terms *report writing* and *clinical reports* to refer to the writing of a range of professional documents about patients and clients. These reports include client/patient notes and records, referrals, professional opinions about clients' needs and management, and program evaluations. The reports can be based on direct assessments of clients or service provision, or on indirect assessments such as those made by staff in radiography and pathology services who review images or samples taken by others. Here we focus mainly on the purposes and types of reports, records, and referrals relating to direct client care or services. We also suggest basic formats and provide advice on effective report writing. Although we focus on clinical reports, many of the issues and strategies detailed are relevant to reports relating to industry clients, school pupils, and other clients outside the health-care system. Chapter 14 provides a different perspective on report writing in its consideration of written proposals for community-health programs.

Purposes of clinical reports

Clinical reports have a number of primary purposes:

- to provide a permanent record of interactions between clients and professional practitioners
- to inform others about the nature of clients' problems and concerns, and about results of assessment or treatment
- to hand over a client to a new service provider
- to direct or recommend how others can or should manage clients' needs
- to request information and services from others pertinent to client management or services
- to advocate for services for a client.

Clinical reports and records store information about clients and about their interactions with professional practitioners in relation to services provided. Such reports and records can be produced for a variety of reasons: for example, recording clinical histories, documenting program needs assessments, reporting on client-assessment results, providing judgements such as definitive or differential diagnoses, requesting additional investigations, making referrals, proposing treatment or service options, providing a second opinion, and documenting recommendations for the client. Reports and records may also summarise or provide regular updates for clients, their insurers, and other professionals involved in health and social services (e.g. welfare and legal services) in relation to the nature and progress of treatment. Ideally, reports provide information in a concise, considered manner. They are a primary mode of communication with other professionals, and sometimes with patients or carers themselves. Referrals may be requests for information or services from other professionals. For example, a speech pathologist may request a full audiological examination for a child whose communication problems and behaviour are consistent with hearing loss; a social worker may request a range of community support services for an elderly housebound person living alone; a general dentist may refer a patient to a specialist practitioner for a complex technical dental procedure.

Across the health and social professions, reports and records can serve many functions, such as informing relevant colleagues, carers, funding agencies, and support systems about professional decisions, recommended services or actions, and service outcomes. The primary goal in writing these reports is to provide information or professional opinions or judgement in a manner that reflects the professionalism and duty of care of the person making the report and serves the interests of the client who is the subject or instigator of the report.

Types of clinical reports

The main types of clinical reports produced by health and social science professionals could be categorised as follows:

- assessments of situations (e.g. concerns, needs, and priorities) and reporting of judgments
- recommendations, proposed plans for action, or management options
- records of progress in the implementation of action plans
- referrals to other professionals or agencies for another opinion or specialist input
- reports on or evaluations of outcomes, achievements, or accountability/budget-reconciliation statements.

Specific examples of these options that are commonly used in the health sciences are listed in Table 12.1.

Table 12.1   Types of clinical reports in health professions

Type of report	Description
Assessments, initial evaluations, diagnostic reports	These record the results of initial assessment of a client's needs, concerns, or presenting problems, together with the professional's judgment (e.g. diagnosis and prognosis), recommendations, or options for action (e.g. program or management plan) and for input by or referral to other professionals to obtain additional relevant information or advice. These reports may be sent to the referring agent or a summary may be provided in a letter back to the referring agent.
Summaries, interim reports, progress reports	These record intervention and progress to date, issues or concerns that have arisen, and recommendations for future action. They are often written for team meetings or case conferences, or for government departments or insurers to obtain ongoing funding for professional services.
Clinical notes, progress notes, charts	These record the results of daily, weekly, or intermittent treatment sessions, and may be kept in departmental client files or in the central record, depending on the policies of the facility. Progress notes are an essential part of larger client records.
Client records	These may form part of a client's main record/management file, which is centrally located but accessible to all service providers and may be kept within a departmental file (e.g. allied health departments in hospitals may maintain separate files that contain details about treatment programs, as well as writing summaries in the client's main record or chart). Psychologists, private practitioners, and social workers would keep individual client case files. Records may be in narrative and/or point form and may include diagrams or charts that present data for treatment goals or outcome data. They typically include relevant images and diagnostic test results. Increasingly, these records are computerised.
Discharge reports	These record the content and outcomes of treatment of or services to a client, reasons for discharge, and recommendations for future management if required. They form part of a main record, and may be sent to an insurer or given to clients and their families for future reference by them or by other professionals.

Table 12.1 Types of clinical reports in health professions (continued)

Type of report	Description
Referrals	These are written to another professional to request assessment and recommendations for management of a client, or to request a second opinion if a health professional or a client is unsure about a diagnosis or prognosis, or is uncertain of the best way to proceed with treatment.
Medico-legal reports	These are requested by insurers, courts, or government departments to provide an independent assessment of a person's current and potential future capacity, or a professional judgment of another professional's work.
Prescriptions	These are a common form of communication between a health professional (usually a doctor or dentist) and a pharmacist or the provider of a specific service or appliance. The information includes the name of the therapeutic agent, dosage and timing instructions, specific instructions on usage, and warnings in case of problems arising.

Formats of clinical reports

The format for a report or record depends on its type and function. Reports on initial assessments of clients need to document all relevant information, provide a summary of assessment results, and list recommendations for future management. Reports that summarise the nature and outcomes of a treatment program need not reiterate all the information from the initial assessment; in such reports it is more important to record the rationale for the program of management, the nature and frequency of treatment, strategies that have proved successful and unsuccessful, and results and outcomes. Referrals requesting radiology or pathology services tend to be brief; referrals requesting clinical assessment by a colleague in another discipline are often quite formal. In order to maximise the chance of an impartial assessment, such referrals provide just enough information to help the professional prepare for the evaluation without predisposing him or her towards a particular view of the nature of the client's problems. Referrals usually indicate the reason for the request and the specific information that is sought. Some reports are compiled by multidisciplinary teams (for example, in aged care facilities).

One of the biggest challenges in writing reports is to provide information succinctly. Students at university may be encouraged to write long, detailed, and comprehensive reports. However, some professions and people in many work settings do not favour long reports. For example, an occupational therapist working in a public hospital may have to comply with a two-page limit in writing an informative assessment report on a child. A professional might document considerable detail in a report designed for publication, but will record only key information in ward notes. Health professionals need to be able to write both short and long reports and to adapt to the requirements of the reader and the work setting. Reports for non-professionals and clients need to be written in language that will be understood by those who read or use them in some way.

Assessment, initial-evaluation, or diagnostic reports

Different disciplines and service facilities have different requirements for assessment reports. For example, medical diagnostic reports following the initial evaluation of a new patient tend to follow a standard structure that includes:

- relevant history and background
- the results of formal assessment
- the results of informal assessment
- clinical observations or impressions
- a summary
- a statement of the problem and a provisional diagnosis
- tests to be ordered (if relevant)
- the prognosis (if possible and appropriate)
- the goals of management
- recommendations for immediate treatment or longer-term management of the patient.
Such medical reports may provide the basis for immediate in-patient management. They will be sent to the referring health professional, and may also be sent to other professionals with a letter requesting additional assessment or treatment. Such reports may also be given to clients for their information. Reports from different professionals and in different situations (e.g. a health-promotion program rather than acute care) have different emphases and content. One of the goals for students in professional education is to learn about the expectations and norms of their specific professional group (e.g. content, form, and lines of reporting) and how to interact and communicate with other professions.

Summaries of care/services, interim reports, and progress reports of services to individuals and groups of clients

Third parties, such as insurance companies and government agencies, frequently require reports on progress, services, treatment, and outcomes. For example, a physiotherapist treating a patient with injuries arising from a motor-vehicle accident will need to provide the insurer with regular reports that not only give updates on treatment and progress but may also request and justify additional treatment. An occupational therapist working with a veteran who has self-care needs will need to do the same for the Department of Veterans' Affairs. A speech pathologist in private practice working with a child with impaired communication may agree to provide a summary report of therapy at the end of each school term, so that the teacher and speech pathologist can plan collaboratively for activities for the child in the classroom in the next term. Community workers will be required to provide progress reports to the organisation providing the funding for their drop-in centre for unemployed youth.

Progress reports tend to follow this format:
- diagnosis, or statement of problem requiring treatment/intervention/service
- summary of previous treatment or services (if applicable)
- description of current services being provided or program being implemented:
  > rationale
  > description
- outcomes/feedback from client
- factors facilitating and/or impeding progress
- strategies found to be effective
- recommendations (and rationales) for:
  > continued treatment, management, or services
  > discharge from treatment or discontinuation of services, or
  > alternative management or referral to another site, professional, or agency.
Doctors frequently have to complete certificates to provide information about a client's absence from work, university, or school. While these are a form of treatment summary, it

may be inappropriate to include a specific diagnosis in them; the emphasis will be on an estimate of the degree of incapacity and the likely time needed for recovery.

Client records

Professionals in the health and social sciences have an ethical and legal obligation to keep an up-to-date record of all contacts with each of their clients. For in-patient settings this is generally called the medical record or patient file. The medical record is the repository of a wide range of documents concerning the patient. It is likely to include a range of assessments, treatment plans, test results, progress charts, and referrals from a number of clinic or in-patient visits. The purpose of these records is to keep everyone involved in the management of the patient up to date with observations and treatments, so that management can be coordinated. These records also provide permanent documentation of patient care and management.

Progress notes

Because of the large number of people typically involved in caring for in-patients, progress notes, or entries to patient records, are kept short. They contain only pertinent information and are written in a factual, non-narrative style. The format of patient records may need to follow set requirements or broader guidelines determined in a given workplace. Figure 12.1 provides an illustration of an entry in a patient record by a nurse using a problem-focused approach.

Figure 12.1 Example of a nurse's entry in a patient chart

30/5/03   1015am Nursing entry

Patient complained of feeling hot and sweaty.
Day 2 post right hip replacement.
Temp: 38.5°C orally. Flushed appearance to face and neck, diaphoretic.
Wound—no sign of redness or oozing. Chest—no cough, normal breath sounds.
IV site—no redness. Indwelling urinary catheter draining cloudy, dark-yellow urine.
Dip-stix urine test—ph 7, + blood, ++ protein, +++ nitrites, +++ leucocytes.
No abdominal pain.
RMO notified. Will come to see patient. Catheter specimen of urine collected and sent to the lab.
Increase oral fluids to 200 ml per hour if tolerated.

Charts

The array of numerical information associated with clients lends itself to charting or graphing. In-patient charts often require specialist knowledge and skill to decipher, as they include sections that chart various physiological functions, usually over time. For example, graphs of temperature, weight, range of movement of a joint or limb, and time taken to swallow a thickened fluid are common. Charts and graphs are the most efficient ways to record (and access) some types of information; they draw attention to trends and significant changes. Dental charts of teeth and oral tissues (recorded as maps) are vital records, updated on the basis of ongoing treatment. Health professionals become adept at using numbers, letters, abbreviations, technical terms, graphs, and a variety of symbols and colours to chart patient progress. Some charts are a permanent part of the medical record that must adhere to a particular format, and the data recorded should not be altered. Other charts are created in response to need, as when a nurse creates a diagram to capture small but significant changes in a wound over a short time. This chart would not be retained as part of the permanent record because the information would be summarised elsewhere. Charts, together with brief records, can be a succinct but powerful way of conveying information to others and of monitoring progress towards goals.

Increasingly, in in-patient settings, charts called *clinical pathways* are used. Pathways are standardised multidisciplinary plans of best clinical practice for specified groups of patients with a particular diagnosis, procedure, or symptom. Pathways aid the coordination and delivery of high-quality, evidence-based care. When you are charting with clinical pathways, you must note any deviations from the expected timeline, which are known as variances. Variance documentation and analysis consists of three parts:

• the variance itself
• the reason for the variance, usually coded by a causative or source category
• an action plan to address the variance and return the patient to the clinical pathway timeline (Badger 1997).

Discharge or final reports

Planning for patient discharge from health care and planning the termination of programs of social services (e.g. welfare services) are both important for a number of reasons, such as client education for self-help, planned transition to home or another less monitored environment, and organisation for follow-up or support from community services. For example, discharge planning for in-patients returning home assists them to arrange for the care they need following a hospital stay. Ideally, discharge planning begins early so that patients and their relatives can consider their options. Discharge planners help to arrange services such as home care, nursing home care, rehabilitative care, out-patient medical treatment, and other help. In developing a discharge report, a health professional may need to assess:

• treatment regimens: current and future medication or treatment needs and their availability
• follow-up physical health care: access to suitable health-care support
• residence: the suitability of the current residence
• follow-up community care: the availability of resources to support the person in the community (e.g. home help, meals-on-wheels, day care)
• activities of daily living: the person's level of competence and confidence for self-care, and the availability of help
• employment, education, financial assistance, and other needs.

Discharge reports typically summarise this information under the following headings:

• Management/treatment goals (including rationales)
• Outcomes
• Issues in management
• Reasons for discharge
• Ongoing needs and problems (if applicable)
• Recommendations for future management

Ideally, a discharge report should provide evidence that discharge has been discussed with and understood by the patient and/or their family. Statements of ongoing needs, problems, and recommendations should incorporate patient perspectives.

Referrals

Referral correspondence can be termed 'writing a referral (letter)' or 'requesting a consultation'. In general, such action is taken when the practitioner(s) currently managing the client's case or providing social services recognises the need for the advice of another practitioner or agency. For example, a member of another profession, a specialist, or some agency or service group may be needed to provide supplementary services (e.g. home care).

A referral letter should provide sufficient information for the practitioner or agency being consulted to understand the client's needs and the requested advice or assistance. The letter should, for example, state more than simply 'Please treat Mr Y. for his (condition)' or 'Please assess this patient, who stutters/limps/is deaf.' The first example provides no information from the referrer that might be useful in understanding the nature of Mr Y.'s condition and his previous contact with health-care providers. The second example fails to provide any background information about the patient that might help the next health professional to prepare for the assessment, and it does not indicate what the referrer would like done after the assessment.

HANDY HINT ☞ **12.1   What to include in a referral letter**

A referral letter should state:
- the nature of the referrer's current contact with the client
- a summary of evaluations and treatment or services received to date (if any)
- test results or evaluation findings if available
- the referring practitioner's professional judgement, opinion, or assessment of the situation
- the reason for referral
- the intended use for any information requested: does the referring agent want the information from the assessment to confirm a provisional diagnosis? to help plan a treatment program? to decide on a management plan for the patient? to request that the management of the patient be taken over? Will services from the agency be provided for the client?

Medico-legal reports

While any document written by a health or social science professional can become evidence in a court following a subpoena, particular care needs to be taken with the preparation of medico-legal reports. To write such reports, you need to have knowledge of report conventions, experience in preparing them, and a degree of professional expertise. Because you may be called to court to defend your report or judgement, you also need a high degree of confidence in your knowledge and professional expertise. Most organisations have a policy on who can prepare medico-legal reports, so if you receive a request to write one, consult your supervisor or departmental manager. It may be someone else's job, or you may be asked to submit your draft report to your supervisor/manager for critique. It may also be shown to the facility's lawyers before a final version is sent to the person who requested it. As a student you should not write any such report without consultation with and approval from your supervisors, as they, not you, are generally legally responsible for your actions.

The guidelines for writing medico-legal reports are in fact no different from those for writing other assessment reports, but extra care needs to be taken to ensure that you can defend and justify every comment made should you be called on to do so. Medico-legal reports tend to contain similar headings to normal assessment or evaluation reports. What makes them different is their increased reliance on quantitative measurement and their decreased use of clinical impressions and observational data. Where clinical impressions and observational data are required to provide a complete picture of a client's functioning, care should be taken to present these as opinions, impressions, and observations. Any inferences or generalisations drawn from such data need to be stated carefully. Guarded expressions such as 'Mrs D. appeared to be ...' rather than 'Mrs D. is ...' are common, as are expressions such as 'Mr M. reported that he can ...' rather than 'Mr M. is able to ...'.

Ethical and legal issues

Many professions have a code of ethics that states how their members should behave towards clients, colleagues, and students. These codes of ethics are typically structured around principles of:

- beneficence: doing good for others
- non-maleficence: avoiding harm (e.g. not providing treatments that are not proven to be beneficial)
- veracity: being truthful (e.g. not telling clients things about their condition or prognosis that are not true)
- fidelity: fulfilling promises (e.g. providing the services to clients that you say you will provide)
- justice (e.g. ensuring equity and access to services for all clients).

Our ethical and legal responsibilities mean we need to act with due consideration of duty of care, informed consent by the client, confidentiality, and ethical principles.

Health professionals aspire to demonstrate ethical behaviour not only in direct contact with their clients but also in what they write about them and how they manage documents about clients. For example, it would be unethical to write in a report that 'Mrs P. is hopeless at doing prescribed exercises and should not receive any further treatment.' Such a statement could violate the principles of non-maleficence and justice.

There are also legal constraints on what professionals can write in and do with documents about patients and clients. For example, privacy legislation provides tight safeguards for *who* can know *what* about clients, and who can gain access to or be shown client reports without the client's consent. *Freedom of Information* (FOI) legislation stipulates that under certain conditions clients can have access to their files. These legal safeguards help to ensure that what health and social science professionals write about their clients is valid and fair. It is beyond the scope of this chapter to discuss all the legislation pertinent to client reports, records, and referrals. However, the following list shows the legislation that bears directly on health and social scientists' written documentation:

- Freedom of Information legislation
- Commonwealth Privacy Act 1988 and Privacy Amendment (Private Sector) Act 2000
- Disability Services Acts
- Medical Treatment Acts
- Mental Health Acts
- National Health (Pharmaceutical Benefits) Regulations 1960
- Health Records Act
- Child Protection Acts

We encourage you to be familiar with these Acts. They differ from state to state (and country to country). You should be directed to specific documents during your course. We next consider some particular ethical and legal requirements that affect the preparation and management of documents about clients.

Duty of care

Implicit in professional codes of ethics and explicit in some legislation is the concept of duty of care. Ensuring the safety of both clients and the public is essential in fulfilling our duty of care. In the context of documents about patients, duty of care implies not writing anything about clients that may cause them harm or deny them access to services. We have a duty of care to provide correct and relevant information in client documents. We must comment and advise only within our area of expertise. We are expected to maintain the confidentiality of information disclosed to us by patients and to keep sensitive documents secure.

Information management

In response to legislation, most human service organisations have established policies on how information about clients is to be managed. In each new setting in which you work, you will need to understand the organisation's particular information-management policies. How should reports and records be managed? Who has access to them, and under what conditions? Such policies generally state the conditions under which documents about clients can be used by six major stakeholder groups:
- patients/clients
- human service professionals
- human service managers
- government and policy-makers
- researchers
- educators and students

The trend towards electronic record-keeping makes information management an even more important consideration for health professionals.

Informed consent

You can only access and share information about clients if you have obtained their informed consent to do so as part of the provision of services to them. At a client's first contact with a health-care service or provider, informed consent should be obtained from the client, the family if the client is under age, or a legally appointed guardian if the client is not competent to provide it. You must ensure that consent is truly informed; that is, you must ensure that the client or the guardian understands the nature of the investigations and services proposed. Valid consent is:
- freely given
- informed (i.e. clients are fully aware of the potential positive and negative consequences of their decision)
- specific (i.e. it pertains to a specified course of action, assessment, or treatment).

Obtaining informed consent from people who are seriously ill or mentally, linguistically, or cognitively impaired (because of, for example, aphasia following a stroke or intellectual impairment) is a challenge. Adapted consent forms that use pictures or symbols as well as text can help in obtaining informed consent (Hersh & Braunack-Mayer 2000).

You must also obtain informed consent from your clients or their guardians regarding who can receive copies of your reports about them, and from whom you may request reports or other information. If you are asked for a report about one of your patients or clients, it must not be provided without informed consent, unless, of course, the request for information is in the form of a subpoena, in which case the report must be provided at short notice. Again, students must check with their supervisors.

Confidentiality

Confidentiality is a key principle in human services. It entails that we must at all times keep information about clients private. We share information only with those authorised to access it; we do not gossip about our clients or talk about them in public places; we safeguard their files.

Ownership of information

It is not always clear who owns a client's file. Is it the client? the professional? the hospital, workplace, health services agency, or community centre? someone else? In some cases, if a report has been requested and paid for by a third party, they are generally understood to own the report. For example, a medico-legal report commissioned by an insurer may be owned by the insurer; the client and other health-care providers may not have access to the report (even though it may be in the client's file) without permission from the insurer. As a general rule, documents about clients in public facilities are owned by the facilities, but clients are entitled to consult them. Sometimes organisations consider that unfettered access to documents may not be in a client's best interest; for example, reports on mental health status may be seen as unsettling to a client. If clients ask to see their file, you need to ascertain why they wish to do so and seek advice from a supervisor before handing it over. In some facilities, clients need to fill out a 'Request for file access' form. Clients can, of course, use FOI legislation to gain access to documents pertaining to them, should organisations restrict access.

So far in this chapter we have discussed the purposes, types, and formats of clinical reports, and some of the ethical and legal requirements pertaining to the management of documents about clients. The preparation of documents requires sound writing skills. Below are some key strategies for successful report writing.

Tips and strategies for successful report writing

Good reports are well structured and provide sufficient detail without being long-winded or containing redundant information. The formats for different types of documents provided earlier in this chapter will help you produce an appropriate framework. The length of

12.2 Writing effective clinical reports

- Use the accepted structure for the type of report in question.
- Write clearly, legibly, and succinctly.
- Provide adequate and accurate information.
- Write at the language level of the intended reader.
- Avoid jargon.
- Use only accepted abbreviations.
- Use correct spelling and grammar.
- Proofread what you write.
- Sign and date reports.

HANDY HINT

Table 12.2   Key strategies in report writing

Strategy	Poor example	Good example
1. Distinguish between opinion and fact.	Susan is a loner.	Susan appears to have a limited social network. *or* Mrs M. reported she is a 'loner'.
2. Use definite, specific, concrete language; give examples.	Peter has no social skills.	Peter does not maintain eye contact, take turns in conversation, or stay on topic. He stands too close to the person with whom he is talking.
3. Use positive rather than negative language.	Eating a normal meal is not permitted until …	Patients can eat a normal meal when …
4. Avoid sweeping statements and over-generalisations.	Like most teenage mothers, Kate is a poor parent.	Kate reports she lacks confidence in her skills as a parent.
5. Use commands if writing instructions (e.g. for medication or exercises).	These exercises should be done prior to meal times.	Do these exercises before eating.
6. Do not use abbreviations or acronyms without first using terms in full and/or supplying a glossary.	The CELF and the PPVT were administered.	The Clinical Evaluation of Language Functions (X edition, year of publication) and the Peabody Picture Vocabulary Test (Y edition, year of publication) were administered.
7. Use vocabulary suited to the reader.	(In a report to the parents of a child with a head injury) John sustained damage to the inferior sulcus of the medial edge of the left parietal lobe.	John's head injury has damaged the left side of his brain in the area that controls …
8. Do not criticise other people or the client.	The doctor who delivered this baby obviously allowed the labour to proceed too quickly.	Mrs B. reported that Emma's birth was 'very quick'.
9. Coordinate ideas.	Jenny said her first words at 12 months of age. She began to use two-word combinations at 18 months of age. By 2 years she was using small sentences.	Mrs F. reported that Jenny began using single words at 12 months, two-word combinations at 18 months, and three- to four-word combinations at 2 years of age.

Table 12.2 Key strategies in report writing

Strategy	Poor example	Good example
10. Use personal pronouns appropriately.	(a) The examiner noted that.... (b) The client said	(a) I noted that Michael ... (b) He said that ....
11. Do not use colloquial expressions.	Janie wore a groovy coat to the interview.	(If it is appropriate to comment on the client's clothing) Janie wore clothes that indicated her interest in fashion.
12. Do not use qualifiers.	(a) Mrs W. was very weepy. (b) Susie was rather withdrawn.	(a) Mrs W. cried frequently during the interview. (b) Susie did not initiate interaction with me, nor did she respond when I attempted to engage her in conversations.
13. Choose short, familiar words.	We will commence this test by ...	We will start your test by ...
14. Use tense appropriately. Use past tense:		
(a) for all past events	(a) Six years ago David is injured.	(a) David sustained a right frontal lobe injury in 1998.
(b) for indicating information that was reported to you	(b) David tells me he has memory problems.	(b) David reported that he still had difficulty remembering the names of friends.
(c) For reporting performance in testing	(c) David names all the items.	(c) David named all the items.
(d) For indicating your interpretation or inference	(d) When I test him, David seems confused.	(d) David seemed confused.
Use present tense for ongoing conditions	David did not read.	David does not read.

the report should be appropriate to the audience. Most organisations prefer reports to be no longer than two pages, although longer reports are appropriate in some circumstances. For example, reports from psychologists, social workers, medical practitioners, speech patholo- gists, and occupational therapists that provide details of formal testing, clinical observations, recommendations for treatment by other health professionals, or classroom programming by teachers may well be longer than two pages. Similarly, medico-legal reports that provide details of assessment and then justification for professional opinions may need to be lengthy. Requests for medico-legal reports also generally come with specified headings, the responses to which may require a longer report.

Reports should provide all the necessary identifying and contact information of the client and the person preparing the report, and must be dated. Reports should be written as soon as possible after contact with the client, to ensure that accurate and current information is recorded. The vocabulary should be appropriate to the target audience. Although technical vocabulary may be appropriate when you are writing to professionals in your field, it is not appropriate when you are writing a report for the parents or family members of a client.

Successful report writing shows evidence of attention to matters of content and style. Use short sentences and plain English (use the plain English websites in the Further Reading section as a guide). Table 12.2 shows some key report-writing strategies and provides good and poor examples of each.

Drafting, proofreading, and obtaining feedback on your reports

Writing professional reports can be a challenging activity. It requires the ability to interpret, critique, synthesise, and summarise a wide array of information and combine it into a read- able whole. It requires you to draft and proofread your report and obtain feedback on its content and appropriateness, perhaps several times, to ensure that it meets the needs of the intended audience. Lovatt (2002) advised health professionals to tailor the readability of their reports to the language levels of intended readers. Given that the average reading age of adults in the Western world is 10–14 years (Vahabi & Ferris 1995), the majority of professional reports would probably be difficult to read for many of our clients, even if free of jargon. A number of readability indices are available, including the Flesch readability test, which is incorporated into major word processing packages. This test includes measures of sentence length, multisyllabic word use, and grammatical features that add complexity to text.

Conclusion

A well-written report is a pleasure to produce and read. We hope the information and strategies in this chapter encourage you to develop your skills in this crucial aspect of professional practice.

References

Badger, K. A. 1997, 'The needs, uses and issues surrounding computerised variance analysis', *Nursing Case Management*, vol. 2, no. 2, pp. 51–4.

Hersh, D. & Braunack-Mayer, A. 2000, 'Uninformed about informed consent? Ethical issues and informed consent in aphasia research', in C. Lind (ed.), *Research, Reflect, Renew: Proceedings of the Annual Conference of Speech Pathology Australia*, Speech Pathology Australia, Melbourne, pp. 126–31.

Lovatt, C. 2002, 'Written communication', in M. Darley (ed.), *Managing Communication in Health Care*, Bailliere Tindall, Edinburgh, pp. 165–203.

Vahabi, M. & Ferris, L. 1995, 'Improving written patient education materials: A review of the evi- dence', *Health Education Journal*, vol. 54, pp. 99–106.

Further reading

Bioethics Website <http://www.csu.edu.au/faculty/arts/humss/bioethic/> accessed 6 April 2004.

Plain English Campaign <http://www.plainenglish.co.uk> accessed 6 April 2004.

Plain Language <http://www.plainlanguage.gov> accessed 6 April 2004.

White, K. 2001, 'Professional craft knowledge and ethical decision making', in *Practice Knowledge and Expertise in the Health Professions*, eds J. Higgs & A. Titchen, Butterworth-Heinemann, Oxford, pp. 142–8.

13 | CASE CONFERENCES AND STUDENT CASE PRESENTATIONS

Ann Sefton and Annette Street

KEY TOPICS

- → What is a case conference?
- → Preparing for a case presentation
- → Getting to know the patient who is to be presented

- → Ensuring that the important issues are included
- → Demonstrating particular clinical aspects (if appropriate)
- → Checking the relevant literature (if there is time)

- → Shaping the presentation to fit the time available

Introduction

Case conferences are meetings in which a patient is discussed, often within a multi-disciplinary team, in order to make decisions about patient management (e.g. diagnosis and treatment). The health or social circumstances of the patient or client are presented for discussion by the group. Students in the different health and social science professions are expected, either individually or as part of a team, to make case presentations about patients or clients and their problems to different groups. For student presenters, the scope of the presentation depends on their stage of development and the particular focus of the conference. The nature of the audience and local customs will determine the specific content and complexity of the presentation; the time available will govern how comprehensive it can be. Presenting a case is a sensitive task, and you must balance the needs of the patient with those of the audience of students and/or professionals.

What is a case presentation?

A case presentation is often the trigger for discussion by the participants in a case conference. Presentations can include interviews with and physical examinations of patients by practising professionals. These skills are essential for making a diagnosis, suggesting lines of investigation, determining progress, and negotiating management. An essential part of professional practice is the presentation of key features of interviews and examinations of patients or clients to a tutor, fellow students, examiners, or a professional team participating in a case conference. A case presentation allows you to demonstrate the processes of clinical reasoning within your discipline.

Presentations range from brief statements that present a diagnostic or management decision, or report on specific aspects of recent progress, to the presentation of information accumulated in more prolonged encounters. Relatively brief oral presentations are widely used to provide concise information to members of the health team who are not familiar with a particular patient or client (for example, in a team meeting, at a change of shift, or in a class tutorial). Written presentations are particularly important for referrals and reports to other health professionals. Because of their central importance in clinical practice, case presentations, oral or written, are often used to assess students.

Preparing for a case presentation

Before starting to interview and examine the patient or client you are to present, you must be clear on what is expected of you. There are often local rules, constraints, or conventions about the length, style, and format of presentations. Most teachers will offer guidelines or models to assist you in developing the relevant skills and will provide you with opportunities to practise. The time allocated determines the depth and breadth of your presentation, and it is essential to organise the presentation to fit the time available.

You should also think about the following factors:
- Is the case to be presented orally, or in writing?
- How much time is available for the prior interview and clinical examination, and for the presentation or conference itself?
- Is it to be based on a single interview or does it reflect a longer association?
- What is the emphasis: diagnosis, immediate management, assessing ongoing progress, or reporting on the negotiation of long-term treatment planning?
- Will the audience or conference members be your tutorial group, a whole class, a professional clinical team, or examiners?
- Will your patient or client be there during the presentation and open to questions from the group?
- Will you be expected to elicit and demonstrate physical signs?
- Will you need to show images or include reports of clinical tests?

- Are you expected to use overheads or PowerPoint presentations?
- Are clinical demonstration aids available to assist you to illustrate your points?

Table 13.1 gives more guidance on how to prepare case presentations.

Table 13.1 Preparing a case presentation

Aspect of case presentation	Possibilities/considerations
Purpose	Diagnostic, procedural, rehabilitative, review
Audience	Peers, senior staff, multidisciplinary team, examiners
Time allocated	Implications for depth and breadth
Resources available and permissible	Access to clinical notes, diagnostic or therapeutic data, or images
Presentation resources	Use of PowerPoint, online case information, overhead projector
Current evidence base	Systematic reviews, clinical guidelines, medication
Patient information available	Single interview, comprehensive work-up, repeat interviews
Patient history	Past health, presenting problems
Diagnosis	Problem statement
Possible action	Active treatment, interventions, or therapies; 'wait and see' approach; referral
Monitoring	Process, timing, plan for review
Outcome	Discharge, continue treatment, cease intervention, or refer on

Each of the health professions has its established patterns for case conferences, emphasising different issues. In addition, there are often local rules about the structure of presentations, and there may be rigid time limits. It is helpful to practise with your tutor or with colleagues before you do a major presentation.

The timing of the conference also influences the nature of the information collected and reported. For example, at an initial encounter in a clinic or hospital setting, the focus is likely to be on taking a history of symptoms and eliciting signs, leading to a set of diagnostic possibilities that might require immediate management or indicate the need for further investigation. At later stages, health professionals engaged in applying diagnostic tests need to demonstrate skills in the acquisition and interpretation of data, and need to offer explanation and reassurance. Once a diagnosis is established, a plan of management must be negotiated, and this requires sensitivity to the patient's needs, values, and constraints. Those providing nursing care, medication, or therapy need to demonstrate that they are able to listen to patients' concerns and offer explanations in addition to applying their specific practical skills.

Establish how much time is allocated for interviewing and for the presentation itself; plan carefully to ensure that the important points are included and are presented in a logical way. You must find out whether you have access to current or previous clinical notes and diagnostic or therapeutic data. Often, however, you must elicit the relevant clinical information from the patient or client without the help of clinical notes, particularly if you are to be assessed. You should take the opportunity to consult the relevant literature, including your texts and sources relating to evidence-based practice. See Case Study 13.1 for an example of a specific case presentation plan.

A medical student presents a patient recently admitted to hospital complaining of severe abdominal pain

Purpose	To demonstrate diagnostic and reasoning skills, based on a single interview and examination
Audience	Peers, tutor
Time	Presentation 8 mins, class discussion 10 mins
Resources	Student's notes of interview and examination
Presentation resources	Whiteboard for discussion, light box for images (if available)
Current evidence base	Evidence-based medicine resources on computer, accessible by student before presentation
Patient history	Report on interview and physical examination, summarising key issues
Diagnosistic possibilities	Presented systematically, in order of probability or of urgency
Possible action	Systematic plan of investigations suggested to exclude key possibilities
Monitoring	Organisation logical, within time-frame
Outcome	Initial diagnostic decision(s), immediate investigation to include/exclude possibilities

Getting to know the patient who is to be presented

In a conference, you will be expected to have a good understanding of the patient or client and his or her problems. It is important to put your subject at ease, even if you are nervous. After introducing yourself as a student, and seeking the patient's consent to be interviewed, you need to outline what will happen. Your patient may prefer to be addressed informally by given name at interview, but at the presentation a more formal title is often appropriate. When you are interviewing children, a parent needs to be present, and for some patients you may need to include a carer or relative. If communication in English is likely to prove difficult, you need to arrange an interpreter beforehand, and you will need to brief the interpreter. If you are expected to review existing clinical notes and test results, make sure that you read them thoroughly beforehand and cross-check important details with your patient.

You may have adequate time to explore issues with the patient in depth. If this is the case, consider 'building' a case history instead of 'taking' it. Building a case history and presentation is based on an information-sharing approach, using a conversational mode to elicit information. You need to combine the emerging bio-medical picture with the patient's view, incorporating psychosocial history into the developing assessment (Haidet & Paterniti 2003). These collaborative processes allow patients to present their views and gain a better understanding of their health problem through explanation and discussion, in contrast with traditional assessments, in which the clinician directs the interview and asks questions that can be answered simply by 'yes' or 'no'.

On the other hand, contact time is often limited, and you may not be able to conduct a leisurely, comprehensive, and systematic review. That constraint creates particular problems in exploring questions relating to sensitive issues, such as the use of drugs or alcohol and sexual practices. When time is short, you need to determine quickly what the key issues are, and

HANDY HINT ☞ **13.1 Effective case presentation interviews**

- Explain your status as a student and gain consent from the patient/client.
- Put the person at ease.
- Explain the purpose of the interview.
- Be systematic and focused in your questioning.
- Encourage the person to contribute personal information and views.
- Keep the language appropriate for the person.
- Explore the necessary contextual information about the person.
- Listen carefully to answers and use them to refocus the following questions.
- Allow adequate time for a considered response from the person.
- Offer information or support if needed.

efficiently acquire as much relevant information as possible. Learn to focus your questions on significant issues rather than aiming to cover every possible aspect of the case, but keep in mind that narrowing too early can lead to errors if you miss relevant information (Maddow et al. 2003). In all cases, listen carefully to the patient's responses, systematically develop some hypotheses as you proceed, and think logically about whether each new piece of information refutes or supports these hypotheses. If you are sure that you have captured the major features, you can then explore additional issues.

You may be required to present a case study of a patient who is unconscious or unable to communicate because of age or disability. You may need to rely solely on written records and diagnostic tests. It is vital that you cross-check important details with other health professionals, preferably those responsible for the test analyses or the clinical notes. You may also need to interview family members to gain a better understanding of clinical and psychosocial issues.

Preparing the presentation

Time limits are normally set for presentations or conferences, and there may be formal rules about the order of information to be given and the use of clinical notes or diagnostic images. The aspects that are emphasised vary across disciplines. It is important to set priorities so that the most important information is presented first, particularly if it is directly relevant to diagnosis or management. You will be able to supply more details, if requested, during or after your presentation.

Providing breadth (an overview of and some context to the patient's background) must be balanced with a more detailed review of the specific problems to be discussed. It is normal to state the patient's name, age, home address, and reason for presenting. The patient's background and occupation are usually also included, as they are often relevant for diagnosis, to understanding the implications of the clinical problem, and for effective management. If you have strictly limited time for presentation, you need to be well organised to ensure that the key elements are included, clearly and logically.

Presenting and discussing the case

After preparation, the next task is to give an effective case presentation. Arrive at the venue early and make sure it is set up the way you need it. Often case presentations and conferences are held in multi-purpose clinical rooms that are rearranged frequently. You may find the seats in an unexpected configuration, or the equipment moved to a new position. Check that the necessary equipment functions properly with your material. If you are anxious about the use of equipment, ask for assistance to test it before the event, or arrange for a technician to help you set up.

You need to know whether the others attending the conference will expect to interrupt you or whether you have a defined time to present. At the outset, briefly explain what you will cover. Set out the sequence of topics, making sure that you link important pieces of information and explain their relationship to each other. Make your clinical reasoning and decision-making processes as transparent as possible. Whether you recommend referral or intervention, your audience needs to able to follow your reasoning. Make clear distinctions between *the evidence* and *your opinion*. Repetition or rephrasing of your key points assists comprehension, as does a clear summary.

As you speak, maintain good eye contact with all the people in the room. You can adjust the speed or content of what you say in response to nonverbal reactions of audience members. Always stand straight and avoid fidgeting and other distracting behaviour. Speak clearly and slowly, especially if you are nervous.

In the discussion phase of a conference, be prepared to handle questions and to intervene if there are misconceptions or errors. Think beforehand about likely issues that might be raised, and decide how you will respond. Treat each questioner and each question with equal respect. If a question has more than one part it is a good idea to list the parts before answering. If you are nervous, jot down a few words to help you remember the various parts of the question. If you are unclear about the meaning of a question, reword it and repeat it to check that you have understood it.

13.2 Interacting with your audience

HANDY HINT

- Be aware of local expectations and rules.
- Arrive early and check the room set-up.
- Briefly explain what you will cover.
- Present your material in a logical sequence.
- Maintain good eye contact with your audience.
- Pace your presentation.
- Watch for audience nonverbal reactions.
- Stand straight and don't fidget.
- Speak clearly and slowly.
- Link important pieces of information together.
- Explain the relationships between pieces of evidence.
- Distinguish between evidence and opinion.
- Repeat and rephrase your main points.
- Provide a clear concluding summary.
- Treat each questioner and each question with equal respect.
- Repeat complex questions to check your comprehension.

References

Haidet, P. & Paterniti, D. A. 2003, '"Building" a history rather than "taking" one', *Archives of Internal Medicine*, vol. 163, no. 10, pp. 1134–40.

Maddow, C. L., Shah, M. N., Olsen, J., Cook, S. & Howes, D. S. 2003, 'Efficient communication: Assessment-oriented oral case presentation', *Academic Emergency Medicine*, vol. 10, no. 8, pp. 842–6.

14 PREPARING A COMMUNITY HEALTH PROPOSAL

Lindy McAllister and Lucie Shanahan

KEY TOPICS

→ Structuring a community health proposal

→ Profiling a community

→ Planning and conducting a needs assessment

→ Preparing a budget proposal

→ Tips for successful proposal writing

Introduction

As governments gradually shift funding from hospitals to community health organisations (McMurray 2003; Wass 2000), professionals in the health and social science professions must become adept at writing proposals and evaluations for community services and health promotion projects. So that health and social science professionals can work effectively in community health teams and in health promotion, university curricula and workplace mentoring programs need to include training in preparing community health proposals and funding applications. This chapter outlines common sections of community health proposals and funding applications, and offers suggestions for writing successful applications. An example of a successful community health proposal prepared by one of the authors is included.

Why write a community health proposal?

Staff in the hospital, community health, and not-for-profit sectors and in community service agencies are all involved in attempting to secure funds for community health and service programs. Proposal writing has become a core skill for professionals at all levels. There'are many possible reasons for writing a community health proposal; for example:

- to increase the quality of a service
- to address an unmet need in your community
- to gain more staff
- to gain more resources
- to develop networks with key stakeholders
- to position your service for increased resources, roles, and funding in the future
- to diversify your work role and add interest to your job
- to gain experience
- to improve your career prospects.

Structuring a community health proposal

Proposals for funds to develop and implement a community service program use similar headings to other funding proposals (see Handy Hint 14.1). In this chapter we concentrate on how to make an argument for your proposal, as the skills involved in doing this are somewhat different from those required for a typical literature review that you might do for a research grant.

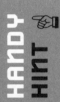

14.1   Structure of a community health proposal

- Executive summary
- Name, details, track record of organisation applying
- Title of project
- Goals and objectives
- Rationale—need for the project, literature review
- Community profile
- Description of project
- Participants/stakeholders
- Strategies/activities
- Budget
- Time-frame
- Evaluation procedures
- Dissemination strategies

HANDY HINT

Note: Not all funding bodies require all these sections.

Making an argument for your proposal

First, you need to review the literature to ascertain whether or not similar projects to the one you are proposing have already been conducted and evaluated. Note the methods of evaluation that were used in previous projects, the credibility and appropriateness of those methods, and the reported outcomes of those projects. A critique of the literature along these lines will allow you to argue for one particular approach to the implementation of your project, and against other possible approaches.

You also need to convince the assessors of your funding proposal that your target community does require the service you are proposing. For example, you would be unlikely to receive funds for a health promotion project addressing the prevention of falls if the target community already has appropriate health promotion activities and services in this area, or if the group you are targeting (in this case, the elderly) is not highly represented in the community in question (say a new suburb full of young families). To convince the funders, you need to conduct a community assessment. This task involves two processes: creating a *community profile* and conducting a *needs assessment*.

Developing a community profile

Creating a community profile is a dynamic process. Communities change constantly and the information you wish to gain from a profile (e.g. demographics of a group within a population) will also change depending on the purpose of your project. A community profile will help you to identify health needs, resources, and potential project partnerships within a community. It involves the collection and analysis of data from a variety of national, state, and local sources. It requires imagination and a willingness to consider all the aspects of a community that are relevant to your proposal, and to consider what constitutes health and wellbeing for that community. You will often need to go to community members themselves and conduct key stakeholder interviews or focus groups to obtain their perspectives on what their needs are. At all times, however, you need to keep in mind that the purpose of the profile is to provide a context for your proposal and a frame of reference for the assessors who will evaluate the merits and feasibility of your proposed program. With the wealth

Table 14.1 Fields and locations of information to be included in a community profile

Key area	Where information can be obtained
Demographics	• Australian Bureau of Statistics (census data): www.abs.gov.au • Local centre of public health • State health department website • 'Echidna' (Victorian demographics information only): www.med.monash.edu.au/mrh/resources/echidna • Completed community profiles (e.g. local Division of General Practice)
Epidemiological data	• Australian Bureau of Statistics • Australian Institute of Health and Welfare: www.aihw.gov.au • Local centre for public health • Local Division of General Practice • Burden-of-disease databases
Environment Local government Recreation and leisure services Health services Industry/key employers Transport	For all these areas: • general Internet searches using Google, Alta Vista, etc., will help you locate specific websites or contact details for these areas (e.g. Shire Council website, local hospital website, sporting club websites, etc.); plan the search terms to use before commencing • review key policies.

of information available on the Internet and the growing number of strategic documents and policies that could contribute to a profile, it is easy to become sidetracked. Table 14.1 lists some typical areas of research needed in preparation of your report and indicates where information in these areas can be obtained.

Planning and conducting a needs assessment

Early work on needs assessment by Bradshaw (1972) is still used as a guide to needs assessment. This work identified four types of need: felt need, expressed need, normative need, and comparative need. Felt and expressed needs are most commonly service gaps or problems identified by people within the community. Normative need is a need determined by experts (that is, what would normally be considered 'right' or adequate for a community). Comparative need refers to past responses to similar issues, or analysis of a similar community's response to the same issues.

It is imperative to determine the type(s) and extent of need in a community and to present this information in your proposal. If a need does not exist, or cannot be argued, the

Table 14.2 Types of, constraints on, and ways to measure community needs

Type	Constraints in expressing or interpreting this need	Measurement
Felt	• People may not ask for exactly what they want for fear it will be 'too much'. • Needs identified may be 'self-based' rather than community-based. • The same problem may be repeatedly raised by the same people. • Opinions can be influenced by media campaigns, such that participants report what they think the researcher wants to hear.	People say what they need: interviews, surveys, focus groups.
Expressed	• Data can be misinterpreted; for instance, waiting list data could reflect a policy decision or a real inability to provide services to all those seeking assistance. • People's beliefs about their 'rights' affect their actions.	Demonstrated by use of services or demand for them: waiting lists, petitions, letters to directors and politicians, etc.
Normative	• This approach is not sensitive to the needs of specific communities. • Professional opinions can change over time. • Epidemiological data can be limited. • Professional opinion may be influenced by political or policy constraints.	Research, professional opinion.
Comparative	• To compare your program with another program, review the parameters (e.g. target group, goals, and activities) of the two programs and the demographics and relevant needs of the two communities. • Superficial knowledge of services in other communities may lead to the erroneous conclusion that these services are superior. A more thorough investigation is necessary.	Investigate programs that have been developed to meet your identified need. Use health promotion databases such as HealthWIZ <http://www.healthwiz.com.au/>.

community will not engage with your program and funding bodies will not fund it. Similarly, if a community's high priority needs are not addressed, the people may not participate in the program because they do not think it is meeting their most important needs. It is strongly recommended that programs not be developed based only on one type of need. Each of Bradshaw's need categories, if used alone, has inherent problems that can be addressed by incorporating the other (felt, expressed, normative, or comparative) needs. Types of need, the constraints of each need, and ways to measure the needs are outlined in Table 14.2.

Developing a budget proposal

One problem noted by reviewers of funding applications is that budgets commonly over-estimate or underestimate what is required. Funding bodies will not fund a proposal that is suggestive of empire-building or seems to be securing resources for other uses. They will not fund budgets that seem to have been 'padded' to obtain more resources than are actually needed for the project. Nor will they fund projects that are likely to be under-resourced and could possibly fail, going by stated goals, desired outcomes, and sustainability. Developing an appropriate budget is a matter of balancing the quality of inputs and outcomes with the quantity of resources available.

When preparing a budget, you must realistically estimate the time and resources needed and obtain accurate costings for items such as salaries, on-costs (see below), transport, facility

---

HANDY HINT ☞ **14.2   Typical items in a budget for a community health project**

Human resources

- Professional and non-professional (e.g. administrative staff)
- Salaries, salary packages, on-costs (e.g. superannuation, workers' compensation, pay-roll tax, casual rates, leave loadings)

Non-human items

- Venue: purchase, rent, or hire on hourly basis
- Building modifications (e.g. for wheelchair access, hearing loops in rooms)
- Insurance (e.g. building, contents, public liability)
- Transport for staff (e.g. fleet, hire, taxis, reimbursement per kilometre, servicing, insurance)
- Transport for clients (e.g. taxis or centre bus pick-up)
- Travel and accommodation costs for staff
- Equipment for office (e.g. filing cabinets, computers, printers, faxes, phones)
- Furniture for clients (e.g. waiting room, tables, chairs, video cameras and players, tape-recorders)
- Tests, toys, books, educational materials
- Consumables (e.g. paper, computer cartridges and disks, stationery)
- Phone and fax: installation of lines, quarterly accounts
- Postage
- Promotion/marketing (e.g. advertising, posters)
- Evaluation costs (e.g. for external consultant, focus group facilitator, statistician)
- Costs of producing and distributing final report

purchase or hire, furniture, equipment, and insurance for cars, building, contents, and people (e.g. workers' compensation and public liability). Don't forget that the salary paid to an individual is only one part of the wages cost for an organisation: on-costs ranging from 10% to 33% (depending on the sector, full-time or part-time status, and so on) need to be added to cover superannuation, leave loadings, long-service leave entitlements, and workers' compensation. Transport costs for staff to travel to meet with clients of the project or for clients to travel to a program centre can be another hidden expense. You need to consider whether you will use an existing car pool, purchase a car or cars (perhaps using fleet purchasing arrangements), hire cars when needed, reimburse staff for mileage in private vehicles, or use taxis, buses, etc. Your manager and staff in your employing organisation's pay office, human resources department, or finance office should be able to help you obtain costings and develop a realistic budget. Items included in a typical budget are shown in Handy Hint 14.2.

Writing successful proposals

People reviewing funding applications often have to read and rank many applications. To catch their attention and avoid being culled on the first read-through, you need a proposal that is well written and well presented, has been spell-checked, meets the granting body's funding criteria, is succinct but still informative, convincingly argues that the project is needed and has a sound budget, and assures funders that successful outcomes and sustain-

14.3   Checklist for writing a successful proposal

HANDY HINT

Does your proposal:
- meet the advertised eligibility criteria?
- fit the specified word/page limit?
- use 'intelligent' layperson's language?
- use accurate figures and quotes?
- use simple subheadings?
- use bullet points to help readers skim?
- look attractive and easy on the eye?

Have you:
- used the active voice rather than the passive?
- grammar-checked and spell-checked your proposal?
- proofread your proposal?
- developed a realistic budget and checked that the budget adds up?
- used the specified font size and type?
- numbered the document's pages?

Will your proposal:
- grab the assessors' attention?
- convince them you can do this project?
- fit into the time-line outlined?
- be feasible with the budget outlined?
- be delivered to the granting body on time?

Source: Based on Galbally 2001

ability will result. Depending on the type of agency to which you are submitting your proposal, and who will be reading it, you may need to alter the type of language you use and the language level. If people outside your discipline or people without a health or social science background will be reading your proposal, you should use non-technical language and avoid jargon. If you are submitting your proposal to a truly community-based agency, some of your readers may have a literacy level below that of university graduates. Your spell-checker can suggest language and vocabulary options pitched at lower levels of literacy.

To achieve these ends you should start working on your proposal well in advance of the due date, so that you can obtain the details you need and write multiple drafts in order to achieve a clear, succinct style that 'sells' your idea. The chances of your proposal succeeding will increase if you ask experienced colleagues to review drafts and you follow their suggestions. See Handy Hint 14.3 for more tips on proposal writing.

An example of a successful proposal

The successful funding proposal in Case Study 14.1 was developed by Lucie Shanahan to obtain funding from a state health department. Guidelines for information to be included in proposals were provided on the health department's website, including word limits for various sections. As you read the proposal, note the definite and positive language used regarding the benefits of this proposed program for the identified community. Aspects of the proposal that made it successful include linking it to existing government-funded initiatives, grounding it in existing literature, and highlighting outcomes across a range of skills and settings. Further, the budget is clear, appropriate, and well argued, and the proposal clearly identifies collaborative networks that will ensure the program is sustainable.

CASE STUDY 14.1

A successful community health funding proposal

NSW BRAIN INJURY REHABILITATION PROGRAM

SUBMISSION FOR PROJECT FUNDING 2003

1. Title of project

Potential Unlimited

2. Unit applying for funding

2.1. Name: XXXX XXXX
2.2. Address: XX XXX XXX XXXXXX XXX
2.3. Contact Person: XXXXX XXXXXX

3. Description of Project

3.1. Brief description of project

Potential Unlimited is a three-stage program that focuses on increasing a person's self-esteem and self-efficacy through the use of experiential education. It was established as an adjustment to injury program for adults with acquired brain injury (ABI), and the positive results of preliminary research into this program warrant further development and adaptation to adolescents with ABI. This project will pilot an adolescent program, drawing participants from across NSW. It will ensure a coordinated delivery of the Potential Unlimited program and provide support to Units as they complete the program. It has been demonstrated that Potential Unlimited does provide an alternative means of cognitive and psychosocial rehabilitation.

3.2. Objectives/desired outcomes

(a)   to support Brain Injury Rehabilitation Program (BIRP) Units and their adolescent clients to successfully complete a Potential Unlimited program
(b)   to foster links with the Department of Employment, Education and Training to ensure transfer of gains from the program to the academic setting
(c)   to secure philanthropic funding to assist in the ongoing delivery of the program
(d)   to provide training to outdoor education staff regarding ABI and its common sequelae
(e)   to identify gaps in the current delivery of the program and develop a resource package for units to assist in bridging such gaps

3.3. Rationale/background

The Potential Unlimited Program was established in 1998 aimed at promoting adjustment to brain injury and increasing participants' self-esteem and quality of life. Current research into this program supports these aims and has proved that the program is a beneficial tool in the rehabilitation and community reintegration of people who have acquired a brain injury. The three stages of the program (group formation/fundraising, Outward Bound course, and follow-up groups) also provide diverse opportunities for targeting and developing cognitive skills, in particular executive function skills. Although initially designed for the adult ABI population, the program can easily be adapted to meet the needs of an adolescent ABI population, allowing cognitive, behavioural and psychosocial intervention to occur in an experiential environment. An abundance of literature (Disinger 1987; Bowling & Williams 1993; Hopkins & Putnam 1993; Van Tunen 1999; Berman & Berman 1995; Anderson 1996) clearly details the benefits of outdoor education programs to adolescents' self-esteem, self-efficacy and quality of life. This program will capture these proven benefits and investigate the use of outdoor education as a means of cognitive rehabilitation. By exposure to a number of activities and environments that require planning, problem-solving, organisational and self-monitoring skills, and by assistance in applying strategies that help with the cognitive demands of these tasks, participants will not only further develop their mastery of cognitive strategies but will also experience success in doing so.

Adolescence is a period heavily characterised by cognitive development, and for many teenagers with ABI already struggling to develop these skills, it is an even greater challenge. This program will provide an alternative tool for paediatric BIRP rehabilitation workers and will create links with school-based support staff to ensure that gains achieved via the Potential Unlimited Program are transferred to the academic setting, in an effort to assist senior secondary school students with the task of completing school. The program is also in compliance with Recommendation 12 of the recent paper by Breust and Associates (2002) that outlined the future directions for the BIRP in NSW. In alignment with this recommendation, this program will foster links with the Department of Employment, Education and Training and will also provide a means of support and information to all paediatric BIRP workers across NSW.

3.4. Proposed Timetable

Strategy	Key Performance Indicator	Time-frame
Appoint advisory group	Group appointed	April 2003
Appoint project officer	Officer appointed	April 2003
Consultation with NSW BIRP Paediatric Workers	Consultation complete	July 2003
Consultation with Department of Employment, Education & Training	Consultation complete	August 2003
Consultation with Outward Bound Australia	Consultation complete	September 2003
Design pilot program & disseminate to key stakeholders	Program designed, feedback obtained from stakeholders, program modified accordingly	November 2003
Design evaluation questionnaire	Questionnaire complete	December 2003
Recruit participants	15 participants recruited	January 2004
Commence pilot program	Stage 1 of program complete	February 2004
Implement Stage 2 of program	Outdoor education program complete	July 2004
Implement Stage 3 of program	Eight follow-up group sessions complete (via telehealth)	August 2004
Administer evaluation questionnaire	Data analysis and final report complete	January 2005

3.5. Evaluation

The project officer will report on a quarterly basis to the NSW Health Department and on a monthly basis to the advisory group. At the completion of the project, the project officer will report on program evaluation received from participants and key stakeholders.

3.6. Impact

Data will be collected to justify the project establishment. The Quality of Life Index and European Brain Injury Questionnaire as used in the adult program will be the tools used for this part of the data collection. They will be administered immediately pre-program, at completion of outdoor education course and 6 months post-program. As well as providing information regarding psychological outcomes, use of these instruments will allow comparative analysis between adult and adolescent programs and respective outcomes. The Cognitive Linguistic Test will be administered at the time of recruitment and 12 months later as an indication of cognitive skills. Surveys of participants, their parents, teachers and rehabilitation workers regarding the functional cognitive skills of the adolescents will also be used to yield evaluation data.

4. Budget

4.1. Total amount sought and proportion of actual cost this represents

Total amount: $19,221.00
Proportion of actual cost: 100%

4.2. Detailed budget breakdown and explanation

Item	Cost	Comment
Capital		
Cognitive Linguistic Quick Test	$494.00	To be used as measure of cognitive gain
Operational costs (chat room establishment, storage, admin. and maintenance)	$1,500.00	E-mail, Internet chat room and teleconferencing to be used for follow-up groups and staff support
Salaries		
Project officer	$12,600.00	Health Education Officer (pro rata 1/2 day/wk for 2 years)
On-costs (calculated at 14.5% annually)		
	$1,827.00	
Other costs		
Travel	$1,000.00	
Training	$600.00	
Program development	$500.00	
Publishing consumables	$700.00	Paper and printing for promotional material, follow-up program booklets, questionnaires, etc
Total	**$19,221.00**	

Conclusion

Because of changes in the demographics of Western societies, together with changes to health funding policies, health and social science professionals increasingly need to take their services outside traditional institutions to communities. Professionals need to understand their communities' needs and preferences for services. This requires skill in needs assessment, networking, negotiating, and team work, to develop funding proposals and deliver and evaluate community health and health promotion programs.

References

Bradshaw, J. 1972, 'The concept of social need', *New Society*, vol. 19, no. 496, pp. 640–3.
Galbally, R. 2001, *How to Win a Philanthropic Grant: The Essential Guide*, Our Community Pty Ltd, Melbourne.

McMurray, A. 2003, *Community Health and Wellness: A Sociological Approach*, 2nd edn, Elsevier/Mosby, Sydney.

Wass, A. 2000, *Promoting Health: The Primary Health Care Approach*, 2nd edn, Harcourt Saunders, Philadelphia.

15

COMMUNICATING WITH THE COMMUNITY ABOUT HEALTH

Linda Portsmouth

KEY TOPICS

→ Understanding health communication

→ Planning and implementing health communication/ education programs

→ Health behaviour changes

→ Face-to-face counselling

→ Mass media health communication

Introduction

Students and graduates in the health and social sciences pass on information about health to their clients or to target groups of people at risk or with specific health needs. Health and social science professionals often ask their clients to change their behaviour or lifestyle in some way. The aim of such requests is to slow or reverse the progression of a health problem or disability, or to prevent a health problem or disability from occurring. Here are some examples that illustrate the diversity of forms of such communication and activity:

- A health promotion professional manages a community media campaign aiming to reduce the occurrence of unhealthy behaviours such as smoking, exercising infrequently, eating little fruit and vegetables, not using sunscreen, and speeding while driving.
- A family-planning nurse advises a 20-year-old woman to use a condom during sexual activity to reduce the chances of contracting a sexually transmitted infection.
- A physiotherapist recommends that a 30-year-old man do certain exercises every day to recover from his injury and return to playing sport.
- A speech pathologist advises the parents of a 4-year-old boy to stimulate his language development by sharing a story book with him daily.
- An occupational therapist advises a 70-year-old woman to use a shower chair to reduce her risk of having another fall in the shower.
- A dietician advises an obese 28-year-old man to reduce his intake of sugar and fat and to increase his intake of fruit and vegetables.
- A general practitioner recommends to a 50-year-old man with liver disease that he stop drinking alcohol.
- An Aboriginal health worker advises women in the community to breast-feed their babies.
- A pharmacist instructs a 40-year-old woman that she must take her new medication with a meal and at the same time every day.
- A drug education worker advises an injecting drug user to use new needles and syringes to reduce the chance of contracting Hepatitis C.

What is health communication?

Health communication is 'the study and use of communication strategies to inform and influence individual and community decisions that enhance health' (National Cancer Institute [NCI] 2002, p. 2). Health communication is not a simple matter of transmitting health information to people who are assumed to be in need of it. It involves the two-way

Figure 15.1 The health communication process

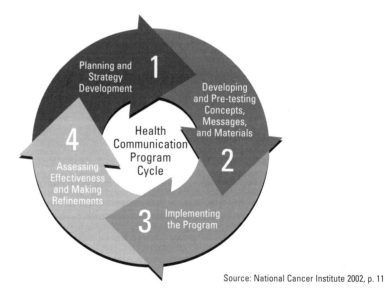

Source: National Cancer Institute 2002, p. 11

flow of information between sender and receiver, as described in Chapter 1, allowing health professionals to develop messages that are understood and accepted by their audience. Human services practitioners need to pay careful attention to feedback from their audience when trying to persuade them to make certain decisions and change their behaviours. Well-planned communication can 'spread knowledge, values, and social norms' and 'initiate change, accelerate changes already underway, or reinforce change that has already occurred' (Piotrow et al. 1997, p. 2).

The health communication process

Communicating to people about health, or 'the health communication process', involves four stages and is circular because, after completing stage four, health communicators are led back to stage one as they undertake 'a continuous loop of planning, implementation, and improvement'. The four stages, shown diagramatically in Figure 15.1, are as follows: '(1) planning and strategy development; (2) developing and pre-testing concepts, messages and materials; (3) implementing the program; (4) assessing effectiveness and making refinements' (NCI 2002, p. 11). There are various activities to be undertaken and questions to be answered at each of these stages to facilitate effective health communication.

Stage 1: Planning and strategy development

In the first stage, you need to clearly and precisely define the health behaviour you are trying to promote and who your intended audience is. It is important to learn as much as possible about the audience and their experience of the health problem (that is, their current attitudes, knowledge, beliefs, and behaviours). You then need to determine if the health behaviour requires new client skills and if there has been an attempt to introduce it before. If there has been, you also need to find out what happened, how the community feels about it now, and why the behaviour is not still being practised.

The communication settings, channels, and activities best suited to reach the audience need to be explored (NCI 2002). The audience may be best reached at home, at school, in the car, at a community event, or in a health professional's office or clinic. Identify when the audience will be most attentive and open to the health message (NCI 2002). The intended audience will find some information sources more credible than others, and some communication channels will be more accessible to them than others. Health information sources and channels that are credible and appropriate to you may not be so credible or appropriate to the intended audience. For example, people aged 35–45 years may prefer to visit their general practitioner and take away a pamphlet to read when they have a health concern. Students aged 14–21 years, however, may search the Internet for answers to their questions about health.

Stage 2: Developing and pre-testing concepts, messages, and materials

The first activity in the second stage is to review materials that already exist. If it is established that new materials must be developed, you need to develop and test message concepts (the main health message), decide what materials to develop, develop them with members of the intended audience, pre-test them with audience members, and then analyse audience responses in order to improve the materials (NCI 2002). This process is essential if you want to produce materials that are easily understood, relevant, and culturally appropriate. Posters and pamphlets, for example, that are believed by the health team to be perfect for their intended audience may in fact be written in language that is too complex, or may contain pictures that the audience will interpret differently than expected. A range of communication channels and methods are described in Table 15.1.

Stage 3: Implementing the program

Successful implementation of the communication plan and program will often entail working in partnership with other health professionals, teams, or organisations. Managing the program involves monitoring activities, staff, and the budget; problem solving; evaluating the process; and revising plans as appropriate (NCI 2002). This phase will also require ongoing attention to maintaining effective group dynamics (see Chapter 22).

Stage 4: Assessing effectiveness and making refinements

The fourth stage involves assessing changes in the audience's knowledge, attitudes, and behaviour in response to the program. Quantitative research is useful for investigating these changes, and involves asking questions of large numbers of people and performing statistical analyses of their responses. Qualitative research commonly asks smaller numbers of people, for example in focus groups, for their reactions to the communication. This method is useful for discovering the reasons behind the initial responses, and is often used in conjunction with quantitative research (NCI 2002).

Commitment is required to initiate and sustain changes in attitudes and behaviour (NCI 2002). The health message usually needs to be repeated and adjusted as the audience's knowledge and behaviour changes over time.

Health behaviour change

Behaviour change also occurs over time. One model frequently used to conceptualise behaviour change is the Transtheoretical (Stages of Change) Model. This model, first described by Prochaska and DiClemente (1984) and summarised by Nutbeam and Harris (1999), describes six stages in the behaviour change process for an individual:

1 Pre-contemplation: the person has not thought about behaviour change.
2 Contemplation: the person thinks about making a change.
3 Determination or preparation: the person makes a commitment to change.
4 Action: behaviour change begins.
5 Maintenance: change continues and health gains are made. There may also be relapse at this stage.
6 Termination: the previous behaviour is extinguished and the person has no temptation to relapse. This stage may not occur for all behaviours.

Using this model, health and social science professionals can design programs to match their clients' readiness to change and help them to progress through the necessary stages of behaviour.

Another useful model used to conceptualise the psychological basis of health behaviour change is the Health Belief Model. This model, also summarised by Nutbeam and Harris (1999), suggests that people are more likely to change their behaviour if they believe that they are susceptible to a problem and that the problem has serious consequences. The model also proposes that people will only decide to change a behaviour if they believe that the benefits of changing outweigh the perceived costs of and barriers to changing. Individuals also need self-efficacy (that is, the belief that they are capable of making the change). Health professionals should therefore aim to communicate susceptibility and threat while promoting the benefits of action and reducing the barriers to action as they arise. In HIV/AIDS education, for example, individuals would need to believe that they are at risk of serious infection and

Table 15.1 Summary of health communication channels, communication activities, and media tools

Channel	Examples of media	Characteristics
Interpersonal	Individual: 　Patient education and counselling 　Instruction 　Informal discussion 　Telephone hotlines	Individual methods can be more credible, motivational, influential, and supportive, and allow two-way communication. Patient education and counselling are most effective for teaching, helping, and caring. However, individual methods tend to be expensive and time-consuming, with limited audience reach. Some can be difficult for certain people to access.
	Group didactic: 　Lectures 　Seminars 　Conferences	Group didactic methods can be best for knowledge transmission and motivation. Lectures and seminars require an effective speaker who has more knowledge than the audience. Seminars are useful for 2–20 people and have the advantage that they allow feedback. Conferences are suitable for professionals and require several authorities.
	Group experiential: 　Skills training 　Behaviour modification 　Sensitivity/encounter 　Enquiry learning 　Peer group discussion 　Simulation/role play 　Self-help	Group experiential methods allow participants to learn via teaching participants through explanation, demonstration, and practice. Behaviour modification is appropriate for the learning and unlearning of specific habits. Sensitivity raising and encounter groups are effective for consciousness-raising. Enquiry learning aids problem solving via group cooperation. In peer groups, members share experiences and support; group members have something in common. Acting of roles can help resolve communication problems and change attitudes. Self-help groups provide peer support and value clarification for therapy or social action.
Organisation and community	Town hall meetings Organisational meetings Workplace campaigns	Community meetings can be familiar, trusted, and influential, providing more support than media alone. Meetings of particular organisations can be inexpensive, offer shared experiences, and reach a large audience. Workplace campaigns can be expensive and might not provide personalised attention, and the organisation may need to approve or change the message.

Table 15.1 Summary of health communication channels, communication activities, and media tools   (continued)

Channel	Examples of media	Characteristics
Low-technology 'folk' or popular media	Story-telling, song, dance, drama (performance theatre and puppetry), and pictures (wall murals, felt or flannel boards, flashcards or flipcharts)	These public activities are the ways people communicated messages to large groups and across time before literacy and the mass media. They are popular because they are entertaining, deal with themes that concern all people (such as love, failure, success, and revenge) and, while based on tradition, incorporate current issues. These methods are most appropriate for age groups and cultural groups that already accept them as an important form of communication. Such groups can include children, young people, seniors, illiterate people, refugees, migrants, and Australian Aboriginal people.
Limited-reach media	Focused information transmission: Pamphlets, leaflets, brochures, information sheets	Focused information methods are better for changing knowledge and attitudes than behaviour, but behaviour change has also been reported. They are better for patient/client education, when content is supported by a health professional, than public education. They are best when there is motivation to change, and are not useful when competing alone against a very resistant attitude. They are more effective with specific content and design features and the use of behavioural strategies. For more information on these features and strategies, see Paul et al. 1997, 1998.
	Newsletters	Newsletters are created for people aligned around an issue who need current information. They maintain continuous communication with the target audience and are personalised. However, producing a newsletter is labour-intensive and requires commitment. They need to be accurate or lose credibility with their specialist audience. They are usually 2–4 pages. They may be in magazine or newspaper format, but can communicate the message without interference from mass-media reporters and editors. They may also be online.
	Videos and audio-cassettes	These media can be instructional and/or motivational. Videos are useful for individuals or groups and can be viewed by an individual or embedded within a group face-to-face session or a website. Audio-cassettes are useful for personal use by adults. (They can be broadcast on television or radio to become mass-reach media).

Table 15.1 Summary of health communication channels, communication activities, and media tools   (continued)

Channel	Examples of media	Characteristics
Limited-reach media (continued)	Agenda-setting, creating public awareness and interest: Posters T-shirts Stickers, badges, drink coasters	These methods can be effective because they use a visual message to appeal to the emotions. They are usually used to support other communication activities. With the use of posters, creative input is required and the possibility of graffiti should be considered. Personalised t-shirts identify the wearer with the health program to cement attitudes and commitment to the program or idea. Stickers, badges, and drink coasters display persuasive, cheap, short messages that identify and motivate the user or wearer and cement their commitment to the program, idea, or campaign.
Mass-reach media	Television: Advertising (paid or public service placement), news, public affairs and talk shows, documentaries, drama (entertainment/education)	Television has the following characteristics: • It reaches the largest audience, and can reach low-income audiences. • The combination of visuals and audio is good for visual appeals and demonstrating behaviours. • Paid ads or programs can reach the audience when it is receptive. • Paid ads allow the message to be controlled but are expensive to produce and broadcast. • Public service ads run infrequently and at times when there are fewer viewers. The message may be obscured by commercial 'clutter'. • Promotion may result in huge demand. • Information may be difficult to retain or pass on. • Some audience participation is possible with a 'roving camera', reality TV, or a studio audience. Mostly there is indirect feedback from the audience via ratings surveys. • Television broadcasts be recorded and used as limited-reach media.

Table 15.1 Summary of health communication channels, communication activities, and media tools   (continued)

Channel	Examples of media	Characteristics
Mass-reach media (continued)	Radio: Advertising (paid or public service placement), news, public affairs, talkback (call-in shows), drama (entertainment/education)	Radio has the following characteristics: • It is cost-effective and useful in creating awareness and providing information. • Radio stations work to a distinct audience, and there is a range of formats for each audience. Many radio stations have few formats that would be useful for health messages. • Radio reaches a smaller audience than TV. • Radio can be interactive (talkback). • Paid ads allow the message to be controlled, are comparatively inexpensive, and can reach the audience when it is receptive. • Public service ads run infrequently and at times when there are fewer listeners. • Information can be difficult to retain or pass on. • Radio facilitates mostly indirect feedback from the audience via ratings surveys. • Radio broadcasts can be recorded and used as limited-reach media.
	Newspapers: Advertising, inserted sections (paid), news, feature stories, letters to the editor	Newspapers have the following characteristics: • Newspapers reach a broad audience rapidly, and provide more thorough news coverage than TV and radio. • News articles can be kept and re-read. • Stories must be newsworthy—that is, have a local angle, be new unique or unusual, be timely and about people. • Small-circulation local papers may take local stories. • Advertising and inserts can be expensive. • Exposure usually lasts only one day. • Article placement requires contacts and may be time-consuming, requiring media releases, interviews, and media launches.

Table 15.1 Summary of health communication channels, communication activities, and media tools (continued)

Channel	Examples of media	Characteristics
Mass-reach media (continued)	Magazines	Magazines have the following characteristics:
		• They have a wide readership and influence. Many specialty magazines reach particular target groups.
		• Magazines have an average life of three to five weeks.
		• They can be useful in a supportive role and to inform and provide social proof of health message.
	Internet:	The Internet has the following characteristics:
	Websites, email lists, chat rooms, newsgroups, advertising (paid or unpaid)	• It is the most adaptable communication medium, as it can provide interpersonal communication (face-to-face via web-cam, personal email, chat rooms), community communication (intranet), limited reach media (newsletters, emailing lists, newsgroups), and interactivity (kiosks, some websites).
		• The Internet can reach large numbers with instantaneous information and updates.
		• Information can be controlled and sites can be designed for specific audiences.
		• The Internet can provide health information in graphically appealing way. It can combine the audiovisual power of TV with the self-paced benefits of print media.
		• Banner ads can direct people to your website. Can be expensive.
		• Particular kinds of software and hardware are required.
		• Not all of the people in the audience have Internet access. The audience needs to be proactive—search or sign up.
		• Newsgroups and chat rooms may require monitoring, and may need maintenance.

Sources: Bivins 1999, p. 126; Egger et al. 1999, pp. 73, 106, 111, 115 & 116; Hubley 1993; National Cancer Institute 2002, pp. 32–3; Newsom & Carrell 1998, p. 381; Paul & Redman 1997; Tucker et al. 1997, p. 285.

that changing their behaviour, by using a condom during sexual activity, will reduce their risk of infection. They also need to believe that this risk reduction is more important than the barriers, such as decreased sensitivity and possible rejection by their sexual partner. Further, they need to feel confident that they can successfully use the condom and have safer sex.

Face-to-face client education or counselling

Client education or counselling, which should include families and carers when appropriate, is one of the most common methods of health communication and an essential aspect of client care. This communication usually takes place during appointments made specifically to give advice or during a one-to-one session with a client. It is also possible to have face-to-face interaction with people who have not yet sought treatment. For example, people may stop at an information display at a suburban shopping centre and ask questions about a health issue to determine whether they are at risk. According to Egger et al. (1999), this is an effective strategy for secondary prevention (reversing the early symptoms of disease) and tertiary prevention (slowing the progress of existing disease). It is, however, labour-intensive and not cost-effective when used for primary prevention, which involves education about risk factors with the aim of preventing disease.

This form of health communication has many positive features. 'The influence of a credible personal source of health information remains strong and should not be undervalued' (Egger et al. 1999, p. 41). Face-to-face communication is interactive, which 'allows better possibilities for success than perhaps any other communication medium' (ibid., p. 42). Face-to-face communication also involves the added dimension of nonverbal communication, such as body language and facial expressions (Hubley 1993). Advice given can be specific to

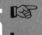

HANDY HINT

15.1 Effective face-to-face individual health communication

- Set aside a place and time at which communication can happen without interruption.
- Greet the patient/client or their family/carer in a friendly respectful way, to put them at ease. Mention that the conversation is confidential.
- Ask about the patient/client's problem and listen carefully to the responses to discover what has been done in the past, what the current concerns are, how much support is available, and how the client feels about the health issue.
- Give relevant, accurate, and specific information in three or four key points. Verbally count them off as they are given. Give the most important information at the beginning. If too much information is given only part of it will be remembered. Take care not to use professional jargon. Repeat important points and then ask questions to check that the patient/client or their family/carer has understood you. Provide written information that can be taken away.
- Help the patient/client or the family/carer to make decisions, being careful not to let your views influence the discussion. Explore alternatives and make sure all issues are considered. Help them make a plan of action.
- Clear up any misunderstandings. Ask the client to summarise the main points of the discussion and the action plan. Let the client know if your perceptions are different.
- Ensure follow-up. Arrange to see the client again, for someone else to see them, or for them to have someone they can contact if they need assistance.

Source: Hubley 1993

the individual and evaluation is easy, as the health professional can ask what the person knows at the beginning of the session and then ask more questions at the end to discover what has been learned (Hubley 1993). Handy Hint 15.1 lists some tips for managing one-to-one health communication.

Face-to-face interactions are not simple when practitioners are asking clients to change their behaviour or lifestyle. Rollnick et al. (1999, p. 3) describe a 'patient-centred' communication style that, while structured by the health professional, follows clients' leads and encourages them to be 'active, vigilant decision makers', in order to help them succeed in changing their behaviour. The authors note that, once a rapport has been established and the agenda set for the interaction, the practitioner then needs to assess the client's readiness for change (as in the Stages of Change Model). The practitioner then needs to gauge the importance of the change to the client: that is, the client's beliefs about the seriousness of the problem and the perceived benefits and barriers to change (as in the Health Belief Model). The client's confidence in his/her ability to change needs to be built up and his/her resistance (that is, the barriers to change) reduced.

Resistance to behaviour change ranges from subtle, silent reluctance to strongly worded rejection. Rollnick et al. (1999) recommend that practitioners do the following things to decrease resistance:

1   Elicit readiness and interest. Ask the clients if they would like more information and ask them which topics they would like information about. Take time to do this and listen carefully to their responses. If the clients do not want information, accept that and do not offer any information.
2   Provide feedback in a neutral, non-blaming, non-confrontational manner. Rather than directly addressing the issues, make comments such as, 'What happens to most people is that …' or 'Many people find that …'.
3   Use language that the client understands and proceed at an appropriate rate for processing and understanding.
4   Give an overall summary before coming down to specific issues.
5   Ask for the client's interpretation of what has been communicated.
6   Use the word 'you' in questions and comments: 'What do you think about…?', 'I wonder how you have been affected by…', etc.

Resistance can also arise if the professional misjudges clients' readiness to change, their perception of the importance of change, or their confidence in their ability to change. It may also arise if the practitioner takes control away from the client. Most people do not like to be told what to do (Rollnick et al. 1999). If resistance occurs, the practitioner needs to reassess readiness, importance, and confidence, and emphasise the client's personal choice and control. Rollnick et al. (1999) suggest that reflective listening (that is, listening and feeding back to clients what they have said to show that they are being heard and understood) is one way to pull back from a situation in which the client feels they are being pressured or controlled.

Mass media health communication

Media or channels (see Table 15.1) are the mechanisms that stand in the middle, between the sender and receiver, in human communication systems (O'Shaughnessy & Stadler 2002). The use of a particular medium can increase the efficacy of health communication to a particular group or community. It is conceptually useful to think of media as either 'limited reach' or 'mass reach' in their communication impact. The mass media use industrialised technology to reach large audiences across distance and/or time (O'Shaughnessy & Stadler

2002). Mass media such as television, radio, newspapers, magazines, and the Internet are all successfully used for health communication.

Mass media effectiveness

Mass media communications can reach large numbers of people rapidly and simultaneously with a consistent message, which is invaluable in the primary prevention of disease and disability. Tied to such communications, however, is the challenge of gaining useful feedback from viewer, reader, or listener surveys. Mass media also cannot carefully target a segment of the audience with a specific health message. The intended audience or target groups are often delineated by risk factors (e.g. smokers or obese people) or demographic groupings (e.g. those with sedentary occupations or parents with young children). These groups are not exposed to any one particular mass media outlet at any one time.

Mass media strategies are useful, however, in presenting general health messages to the whole community, keeping in mind that messages will be perceived in different ways by different people depending on their beliefs about health and the benefits of and barriers to change (Health Belief Model). The impact of health messages will differ at the various stages of individual behaviour change. Egger at al. (1999) report that mass media campaigns are most influential in the pre-contemplation and contemplation stages of the Stages of Change Model. These are the times at which individuals have not yet considered behaviour change or have just considered behaviour change but have not yet become committed to the idea. Mass media work by 'by raising the salience and personal relevance of the issue' (Egger at al. 1999, p. 97). This strategy has a moderate influence at the preparation stage (when a person has committed to change) 'by reinforcing perceptions of self-efficacy and maintaining salience of the perceived benefits of adopting the recommended behaviour'. It is least influential in the action and maintenance stages, when beliefs and attitudes are well established and socio-environmental factors, such as the people directly interacting with the individual, have a greater impact on behaviour (Egger at al. 1999, p. 97).

A well-planned mass media campaign, according to Hubley (1993), can:
- transmit knowledge
- change behaviour—when it is a one-off behaviour (e.g. immunisation) that is not difficult to perform and the community is positively disposed towards implementing it and needs only a stimulus for action
- set the agenda—that is, bring an issue to community attention so it starts to be discussed
- create a general community feeling that supports change
- inform the community about new ideas.

Mass media objectives

The mass media usually aim for individual behaviour change by:
- *informing or educating*: they provide information about negative or positive health effects and clarify misconceptions
- *motivating or persuading*: they reinforce positive behaviour, generate emotional responses about an issue, or make individuals aware of the health issue
- *directing*: public service announcements can direct people to information on where and how to gain assistance or inform them of specific events, programs or services (Egger et al. 1999).

The mass media can also stimulate socio-political change (Egger et al. 1999). Media advocacy aims to create or increase community awareness of issues, create or maintain a positive attitude towards certain healthy behaviours, legitimise a health problem as an issue for community concern, or generate a 'positive community mood' towards a regulatory policy or a research project (Egger et al. 1999). The successful anti-smoking campaigns in Australia are an example of how media advocacy has been used in combination with strategies targeting individuals.

Mass media methods

Egger et al. (1999) describe three major mass media methods:

1 *Advertising.* This is the paid or unpaid placement of advertising messages in the mass media. Examples of this method include television advertisements promoting the QUIT campaign, advocating a reduction of speeding while driving, or promoting osteoporosis assessment. This advertising has in part been a response to the success advertisers have had in using the mass media to promote unhealthy behaviours and products, such as cigarettes and high fat food. In advertising, health professionals have control over content, message exposure, and frequency of exposure to the target group (i.e. when and on what channel it is shown). The major disadvantages are the cost of production and the short exposure time, though, because of the high number of people exposed to the message, the exposure cost per individual is low.

2 *Publicity.* This occurs when the media are attracted to cover a story in news, current affairs, documentary, or lifestyle programs, or when articles in the print media create, maintain, or increase the intended audience's awareness of or support for a health message or organisation. Health professionals may be involved in writing media releases, giving interviews, or giving presentations at press conferences. Publicity can reach large numbers in a short time, but there is less control over the message content, the exposure, and the frequency of exposure than with advertising. It is, however, cheaper than advertising and is perceived as more credible, since journalists are considered less biased than advertisers.

3 *'Edutainment'.* This is the inclusion of health messages (education) in broadcasts or publications designed for entertainment, such as episodes of television dramas and soap operas, and films for cinema release. Edutainment reaches large numbers of people who may not choose educational media programming. Health professionals can ask media writers and producers to insert particular health messages into their scripts. Writers and producers may approach health professionals for advice as they introduce health-based storylines in their scripts. This method can be inexpensive unless health organisations sponsor or produce the programs.

Making mass media successful

Egger et al. (1999) note that mass media health communication campaigns are different from other community-based health programs as they are imposed upon the community rather than a result of the mobilisation of the community. Hubley (1993) noted, however, that it is possible to use the mass media to successfully promote health by understanding the target audience, pre-testing the message, and evaluating media impact.

Mass media audiences are bombarded with stimuli. Human services professionals, often working with media professionals, need to discover the factors that influence the intended audience's selection and perception of health messages. These factors, according to Egger et al. (1993), include:

• mechanical factors that make a message stand out against competing messages (e.g. eye-catching pictures, headlines, and movement)

• psychological factors, as people respond to messages that offer them a benefit that relates to their interests, attitudes, and beliefs

- message factors that make the message as acceptable as possible to the intended audience (e.g. linking the message to an already accepted belief and presenting two-sided appeals that leave the audience to draw their own conclusion rather than tell them what to think or do).

The following types of appeal, seen in advertising, publicity, and edutainment, have been successful in conveying health messages that effectively influenced the intended audience:
- fear appeals, which attempt to frighten the intended audience into action
- humorous appeals, which use humour to gain attention and hold interest
- logical/factual appeals, which convey facts and figures as objective proof of the importance of behaviour change
- emotional appeals, which arouse emotions and paint images in the mind to persuade or motivate the intended audience to change
- one-sided appeals, which present the advantages of taking action
- two-sided appeals, which present both the benefits and the disadvantages of taking action
- positive appeals, which ask for action, that is, for the intended audience to do something healthy (e.g. eat more fruit and vegetables)
- negative appeals, which ask the intended audience not to do something unhealthy (e.g. smoke tobacco) (Hubley 1993).

Conclusion

The key to successful health communication is to work at every stage of the two-way process with members of the intended audience. This is critical if you are to move beyond information transmission to behaviour change communication. Careful consideration of individual factors, such as readiness to change and personal health beliefs, is required for successful face-to-face client education or counselling. The mass media, while they cannot target individuals, can be effective in reaching the whole community with a general health message. Such messages are most effective when they have been developed with and tested by members of the intended audience.

References

Bivins, T. H. 1999, *Public Relations Writing: The Essentials of Style and Format*, 4th edn, NTC/Contemporary Publishing, Lincolnwood, Illinois.

Egger, G., Donovan, R. & Spark, R. 1993, *Health and the Media: Principles and Practices for Health Promotion*, McGraw-Hill, Sydney.

Egger, G., Spark, R., Lawson, J. & Donovan, R. 1999, *Health Promotion Strategies and Methods*, rev. edn, McGraw-Hill, Sydney.

Hubley, J. 1993, *Communicating Health: An Action Guide to Health Education and Health Promotion*, Macmillan, London.

National Cancer Institute 2002, *Making Health Communication Programs Work*, National Cancer Institute, National Institutes of Health, US Department of Health and Human Services, Bethesda, Maryland <http://www.nci.nih.gov/pinkbook> accessed 23 March 2004.

NCI—*see* National Cancer Institute.

Newsom, D. & Carrell, B. 1998, *Public Relations Writing: Form and Style*, 5th edn, Wadsworth, Belmont, California.

Nutbeam, D. & Harris, E. 1999, *Theory in a Nutshell: A Guide to Health Promotion Theory*, McGraw-Hill, Sydney.

O'Shaughnessy, M. & Stadler, J. 2002, *Media and Society: An Introduction*, 2nd edn, Oxford University Press, Melbourne.

Paul, C. L. & Redman, S. 1997, 'A review of the effectiveness of print material in changing health-related knowledge, attitudes and behaviour', *Health Promotion Journal of Australia*, vol. 7, no. 2, pp. 91–9.

Paul, C. L., Redman, S. & Sanson-Fisher, R. W. 1997, 'The development of a checklist of content and design characteristics for printed health education materials', *Health Promotion Journal of Australia*, vol. 7, no. 3, pp. 153–9.

Paul, C. L., Redman, S. & Sanson-Fisher, R. W. 1998, 'Print materials as a health education tool', *Australian and New Zealand Journal of Public Health*, vol. 22, no. 1, pp. 146–8.

Piotrow, P. T., Kincaid, D. L., Rimon, J. G. & Rinehart, W. 1997, *Health Communication: Lessons from Family Planning and Reproductive Health*, Praeger, Westport, Connecticut.

Prochaska, J. O. & DiClemente, C. C. 1984, *The Transtheoretical Approach: Crossing Traditional Boundaries of Therapy*, Dow Jones Irwin, Homewood, Illinois.

Rollnick, S., Mason, P. & Butler, C. 1999, *Health Behavior Change: A Guide for Practitioners*, Churchill Livingstone, Edinburgh.

Tucker, K., Derelian, D. & Rouner, D. 1997, *Public Relations Writing: An Issue-driven Behavioral Approach*, 3rd edn, Prentice Hall, Upper Saddle River, New Jersey.

PART 3

PRESENTATION STYLES, SKILLS, AND STRATEGIES

16	Text Style and Formatting: Using Styles and Templates	155
17	Preparing Graphics and Tables	161
18	Preparing Posters	169
19	Giving Talks in Class	176
20	PowerPoint Presentations	184
21	Presenting Talks at Conferences	194

16 | TEXT STYLE AND FORMATTING: USING STYLES AND TEMPLATES

Charles Higgs and Joy Higgs

KEY TOPICS

→ Planning your document

→ Using styles and templates

→ Simple style management for essays and assignments

→ Table of contents

→ Using the Outline function in Word

Introduction

Presentation and layout are important in undergraduate reports and papers, and are very important in theses and journal papers. It is valuable to learn strategies and functions that help with these tasks, such as the use of styles to streamline word processing. Functions like styles, automated tables of contents, and templates all make creating your documents easier and allow for greater consistency of layout and format.

A note about versions before you begin: the instructions in this chapter relate to Word 2000. There are subtle differences between Word 95, 98, 2000, and XP. If in doubt about how to do something, you should use the HELP function to find the exact sequences of commands in the version you are using.

Planning the style of your document

Your aim is to produce a scholarly, aesthetically pleasing document, with consistent formatting throughout that is appropriate to the discipline in which you are writing and to the genre of the article (e.g. research report, essay, poster, story, conversation piece). Before commencing writing, you need to:

- decide upon the basic formatting that you will use throughout the document
- make sure you are familiar with the basic features of your word processing software (for example, do you know quick and easy ways to select text, move around your document, add tables, format text, and indent?)
- practise inserting figures, tables, etc., between text and moving them around, to minimise difficulties in the final stages
- understand how to use styles.

Thesis style

Talk to your supervisor about what your university or college expects with regard to the layout of a thesis. You need to consider aspects like the margin size needed for binding of a thesis. Your university will probably have this information on its website. Other aspects include whether special paper (e.g. acid-free or archival paper, or picture quality paper if using coloured graphics) will be needed and whether the binding needs to be temporary or permanent. Remember that the style of the whole package is important, as well as the content.

In planning your thesis's style, you must make decisions in relation to the following matters (see also Chapter 9):

- Font: serif or sans-serif (compare Times New Roman and **Arial**), size 11 or 12 point for main text.
- Page set-up:
  - > Margins: allow for binding and variations in landscape and portrait layout.
  - > Justification: left and/or right (see Table 16.1). There are many ways to lay out your text. Decide which you prefer. Remember to be consistent throughout your document.
  - > Page size: in Australia A4 is commonly used.
  - > Orientation: portrait (vertical) or landscape (horizontal) .
  - > Line spacing: check to see if you are required to use double or 1.5 spacing.
- Page number positioning: be consistent, even if you are using some portrait and some landscape layout. This may require manual insertion of a page number on the landscape pages and automatic page number insertion on the portrait (main) pages.
- Footnotes or endnotes: if possible use the default offered in the software. Sometimes footnotes are not permitted (as in many journals).
- Colour: yes/no.
- Shading: yes/no. If you use shading, make sure your text is readable, especially after photocopying.
- Any additional items: lines, borders, trim, etc. These should complement and enhance the text, not be obvious distractions.

Serif and sans-serif fonts

The small decorative finish at the end or bottom of a letter is called a *serif*. Observe the differences in the following fonts:

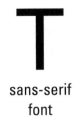

sans-serif
font

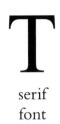

serif
font

The character on the left does not have the decorations and is a sans–serif font (*sans* is the French word for *without*). The character on the right has serifs and is called a serif font.

Generally, serif fonts are easier to read (although there is a degree of personal preference here) because we are used to reading serif fonts in most text (books, newspapers, etc.). For your own paper, you might choose to use a serif font (e.g. Times New Roman) for the body of your work and a sans-serif font (e.g. Arial) for the headings. Figure 16.1 shows some different font sizes in Arial and Times New Roman. Note that the Arial font of the same number is actually physically larger than the Times New Roman.

Figure 16.1   Text sizes: Examples

10 point Arial (sans-serif font)

12 point Times New Roman (serif font)

18 point Arial (sans-serif font)

18 point Times New Roman (serif font)

24 point Arial (sans-serif font)

24 point Times New Roman (serif font)

Table 16.1   Justification of text

Left	Right	Both or full justification
Left justification is good for lists and tables of words.	Right justification can be used for effect or to line up a set of numbers without decimal places or with the same number of decimal places. Use decimal tabs (Shift Tab) rather than right justification in table columns of figures with unequal numbers of decimal places.	Full justification gives a pleasing effect, like a book layout. But watch out for the 'stretch effect' —too much white space. Left justification can be preferable if this is a problem (or you could use manual hyphenation to break up long words at the end of lines). See examples in this book.

☞ **16.1 Switching between different printers and software**

Remember the following points, especially if your work (e.g. a thesis) is being done over a long period of time and/or in different venues:

- Different printers have different page capacities for printing. Your layout (e.g. manual page breaks) may not appear as planned if you design it for one printer and print it out on another.
- Some formatting may not translate well between different software programs (e.g. Word and WordPerfect) or between different versions of the same program. If you are writing the work with other authors it may be advisable to share the developing document in a standard format (e.g. save the file as 'RTF'—rich text format) and then perform a final format. If possible, it is preferable to use the same software throughout the writing of a long work such as a thesis.

Include the relevant decisions in a personal text style that you will put in a template and use when typing content (see instructions below). At a later stage you can easily include additional style items (e.g. additional heading, font, or paragraph styles).

Word styles

When we make a word bold, we change only one characteristic of the word. When we apply a style to a word or sentence in Word we can change an entire set of characteristics at once. For example, if we decide that a heading level in our document should all be bold, 18 point Arial, and centrally aligned, we can apply all the features simultaneously by applying a style with these characteristics. Moreover, if all our headings have been created using a common style and we decide that we want to change the characteristics of every heading to italic, 15 point Times New Roman, and left aligned, we simply apply the changes to the style and every heading that uses that style is automatically modified.

The simplest way to apply styles is to click on the STYLE drop-down list and select the required style. This style will be applied to the paragraph that the cursor is currently in. Word comes with a number of styles that should meet most needs. If you want to apply a style to a paragraph, remember to place the cursor within the paragraph or select the entire paragraph. Styles can also be assigned to selected text (i.e. a word or words) if required, although for one-off situations it is easier to format the text manually. You can also create your own styles (as detailed later in this chapter).

If you apply a style and decide that it is not what you want you can modify it using FORMAT, STYLE. Note that if you want to change a heading style globally you should not reformat the text in one heading only. This will only change the heading being edited, not every instance of the same style.

☞ **16.2 Using shortcut keys**

The basic styles (e.g. Headings 1, 2, 3, etc., and Normal) and most text formatting (e.g. bold and italic) can also be applied using shortcut keys. Select HELP and search for SHORTCUT KEYS.

Sometimes a basic style does not contain the exact layout or font you want. You can modify the style within that document by selecting FORMAT, STYLE, selecting the style you want and then selecting MODIFY. Carry out the modifications you want, then apply them. This will change the style formatting throughout the document. When you next apply that particular style in this document it will have the formatting of the modified style. Try this out by creating a dummy document and practising applying and changing styles.

Changing the 'Normal' style

As an exercise, try changing the main text in a document (NORMAL style). With the document open and your cursor in the body of the text select FORMAT, STYLE. Under LIST show STYLES IN USE. There will be some built-in styles shown, including NORMAL. With NORMAL highlighted, click on MODIFY and then FORMAT, FONT. Select any font and then click on OK. Click OK on the MODIFY STYLE dialogue box then APPLY, to apply the font to all the instances of NORMAL style in the current document. This technique can be applied to any existing style in this document.

16.3   Font survival

For a thesis or report that is going to be opened on another computer you should keep the fonts simple (e.g. Times New Roman and Arial). Unless you embed the fonts (look this up in HELP), you cannot guarantee that your document will look the same on another computer. The same embedding technique can be used to create your own styles. To do this select FORMAT, STYLE but click on NEW instead of MODIFY.

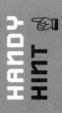
HANDY HINT

Templates

If you want to use the same layout and styles in more than one document (e.g. if each chapter in your thesis is a separate document) you should create your own template. All Word documents are based on a template. When you choose FILE, NEW to create a new document you are by default creating a document based on the NORMAL template. However, if you create your own templates, such as templates for letterhead pages, memos, and a thesis, then each of these options will appear when you select FILE, NEW. Note that templates are stored in the computer on which you are working. If you want to move a template from one computer to another you must copy the template to the second computer.

Creating a simple template

The following steps can be used to create a simple template:

- Open a blank document and create or modify your styles.
- Click FILE, PAGE SETUP and check that paper size is A4. This is important!
- Set the margins. Often thesis margins will be prescribed by your university. If not, make sure that the margin on the binding side remains consistent and sufficient to allow for the binding or for storage in a ring binder, if necessary. The other margins should normally remain consistent, except on pages with landscape tables, which may require narrower margins.
- Set up other features that you want repeated throughout every document based on this template. This may include spelling and grammar, colours, language, AutoCorrect, etc.

- With the document open click on FILE and SAVE AS. Click on the SAVE AS TYPE drop-down list and choose DOCUMENT TEMPLATE. Type in a descriptive name, such as 'Thesis Template' or 'Chapter Template', in the FILE NAME box and click the SAVE button.
- Whenever you start a new chapter use this template. To do this you must use FILE, NEW. Click on the icon or the name of the template; make sure in CREATE NEW that DOCUMENT is checked. Then click on the icon or the name of the template to open it.

Table of Contents

Previously we mentioned the built-in styles, including Headings 1, 2, 3, etc. Not only do these headings allow us to create an aesthetically pleasing document, we can also use the heading styles to create an automatic table of contents. To do this, select INSERT MENU and INDEX & TABLES. Click on the TABLE OF CONTENTS tab. Decide which headings you are going to use in the Table of Contents. Typically they would be Heading 1, Heading 2, and Heading 3, but this will depend on how you have laid out your thesis. Choose OK to insert the table of contents. If you edit the document further you can update the table of contents by selecting the table and pressing the F9 (update fields) button. You will be given the option of updating either the entire table of contents or just the page numbers.

It's a good idea to keep large chapter files separate until the end of your thesis writing, so that you do not lose a lot of work if one file becomes corrupted. However, if your chapters are written as separate files, you will need to combine all the files to create the table of contents electronically. (Your files may be too big to do this efficiently or safely.) You can learn more about combining files by choosing HELP and searching for 'Create a master document'.

Outline view

We typically view a page in either Normal or Print Layout view. Once a document becomes larger than a few pages it is sometime easier to view as an Outline. Select VIEW, TOOLBARS, OUTLINING.

Outline view provides a separate toolbar that allows you to view an entire document or only specific headings in the document. If the SHOW LEVEL box is set to Level 1, for example, only headings styled as Heading 1 can be viewed. You can drag a heading to any location within a document, and the heading (and all the content between it and the next heading) will move to the new position. Headings can also be promoted (e.g. Heading 2 changed to Heading 1) or demoted using the OUTLINING toolbar. You can also change the style of text using the OUTLINING toolbar.

Conclusion

Presentation and layout are important in undergraduate reports and in papers, theses, and journal articles. The features in your word processing software can help you to improve the layout and aesthetic presentation of your work. The features can also make the creation and management of large documents easier and more efficient.

17 | PREPARING GRAPHICS AND TABLES

Charles Higgs and Joy Higgs

KEY TOPICS

→ Forms of graphics and tables commonly used in health and social sciences communications

→ The purposes of these graphics and tables

→ Guidelines for the presentation of graphics, graphs, and tables

Introduction

Graphics are important communication devices. The reader's perceptions of the quality of communication are influenced by the quality of presentation of the text and associated graphics and tables. Graphics include figures and diagrams, pictures, photos, drawings, icons, maps, and so on. There are many instances where images are more powerful communicators than words; they fire the imagination, prompt pattern recognition (e.g. of illnesses) and communicate relationships (e.g. locations, differences in magnitude, rate). They can be used to summarise quantitative information in a visual form that is easier to understand than detailed tables of figures. Graphics can communicate principles and scientific laws (e.g. momentum). Graphics can also entertain and stimulate as part of a presentation.

Tables are valuable means of summarising quantitative data and presenting groups of data, such as variable scores for individual subjects in a research study, different groups' performances on tests, and differences between experimental and control groups. Tables can also summarise qualitative data, such as key components of theoretical models, findings of different qualitative research studies, trends in research topics, and sets of data such as signs and symptoms associated with different diseases.

Effective graphics and tables

To be effective, graphics and tables (Hay et al. 2002) need to be relevant, concise, comprehensible, meaningful as 'stand alone' items without the text, and referenced (i.e. any sources for the data or the graphic must be acknowledged). Tables and figures need clear and comprehensive titles, legends, labels, and footnotes. The format of tables and figures is a matter of convention and preference. Some people argue, for instance, that the title should be placed below graphs and figures and above tables (Price 1997a, b). Check the common practice in relation to assignments or theses in your school, or follow your university's guide to presentation of essays and assignments, or use the style of the journal for which you are submitting a paper.

Graphs

There are many types of graphs, including scattergrams, line graphs, bar charts, histograms, population pyramids, pie charts, and logarithmic graphs. Instructions for constructing all these graphs can be found in Hay et al. (2002). Here we concentrate on three types of graph: line graphs, bar charts, and pie charts.

Many spreadsheet packages can help you to create graphs. The bar chart in Figure 17.1 contains a table of data at the bottom of the graph. By entering these data in your Excel spreadsheet (for example), selecting the data, clicking on the graph icon, selecting the bar chart option, and following the prompts to input title, legends, and so on, you can produce this graph with relative ease. (Note that the guidelines in this chapter relate to Office 2002 software, but

Figure 17.1 Example of a bar chart: Pre-test and post-test scores for groups A–D

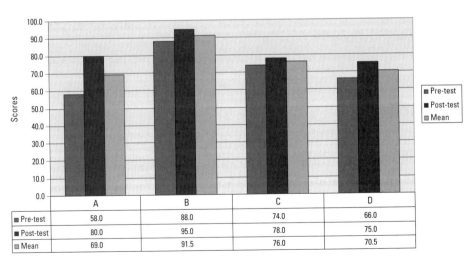

	A	B	C	D
Pre-test	58.0	88.0	74.0	66.0
Post-test	80.0	95.0	78.0	75.0
Mean	69.0	91.5	76.0	70.5

Groups

the processes are very similar in other versions of Office software.) With a reasonable amount of practice you should be able to create and modify charts in Excel from a variety of data sets.

Next we create a line graph using Excel. Look at the data in Table 17.1. The letters and numbers on the top row and left column indicate the cell addresses on the spreadsheet. Select the cells B3 to H6 and click on the graph icon; choose the 'multiple line graph' option and create this graph, adding the title, etc. The result should look like Figure 17.2. Use the data in Table 17.2 to create a pie chart like Figure 17.3.

Table 17.1 Data for line graph

	A	B	C	D	E	F	G	H
1		Test scores on VEM at hourly intervals						
2								
3		1	6.3	7.7	7.4	8.8	7.4	9.5
4	Subjects	2	3.5	3.9	4.4	5.9	7.9	8.7
5		3	5.6	5.7	5.7	5.4	5.9	5.8
6		Mean	5.1	5.8	5.8	6.7	7.1	8.0

Note: The dark shading shows cell references on Excel. These do not appear on the finished graph. The light shading indicates the data area to be converted to a graph.

Figure 17.2 Example of a line graph: Test scores on VEM at hourly intervals

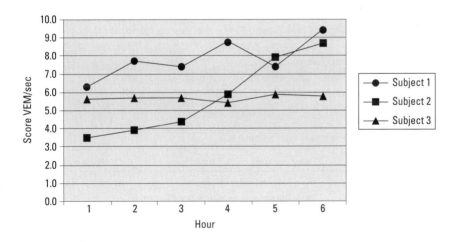

Table 17.2 Data for pie chart: States' incidence of condition X per 10,000 population

	NSW	VIC	NT	QLD	TAS	SA	WA	ACT	AUST
%	16	9	14	10	5	6	19	21	100
n/10K	73	41	64	46	23	28	87	91	453

Figure 17.3 Example of a pie chart: Incidence of condition X per 10,000 population in Australian states and territories as percentage of total incidence

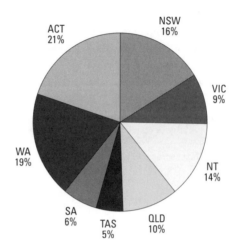

Tables with word data

See Tables 17.3 and 17.4 for examples of tables containing word data. To create a table using a word processing file, take the following steps:

1 Plan your table. This can involve making rough notes or drawing up the actual table on paper.
2 In Word:
   > Click on TABLE, INSERT TABLE.
   > Choose, say, 3 columns and 7 rows (1 for the title and 6 for data).
   > Add the title.
   > Insert and bold the column headings.
   > Add the relevant data/information in each row.
   > Adjust the column widths and spacing to optimise the table.

Table 17.3 Theories of benchmarking: Example 1

Theory	Key content	Reference
Best current national practice	• 3 key indicators measured • Top national scoring hospital identified	Frederickson 1999
Best international model	• 10 key indicators measured • Top scoring unit for each indicator identified	Schmidt & Abrendt 2001
Achievable growth target	• Own unit as benchmark • Achievable growth on indicators set	Wu & Fenwick 2000
Ideal position model	• Use of research data and theoretical models • Ideal position for 6 key parameters set	Trendle 2000

3   Choose your own style for your tables or follow the prescribed style set by your school or the journal you are submitting a paper to. Will you include lines to divide rows and columns? Is shading in tables appropriate and useful?

Table 17.4   Theories of benchmarking: Example 2

Theory	Key content	Reference
Best current national practice	• 3 key indicators measured • Top national scoring hospital identified	Frederickson 1999
Best international model	• 10 key indicators measured • Top scoring unit for each indicator identified	Schmidt & Abrendt 2001
Achievable growth target	• Own unit as benchmark • Achievable growth on indicators set	Wu & Fenwick 2000
Ideal position model	• Use of research data and theoretical models • Ideal position for 6 key parameters set	Trendle 2000

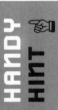

17.1   Working with tables

- Using TAB in tables will move your cursor to the next cell, or create a new row if you are in the last cell in the table. To tab within table cells use CTRL TAB.
- Don't use block (i.e. left and right) justification in tables; it can lead to awkward spacing.
- Align words in vertical columns using left or centred justification; align numbers using right or decimal justification.
- You can resize all the columns in your table using TABLE, AUTOFIT.
- You can automatically format a table to a variety of styles using TABLE, TABLE AUTOFORMAT.

Tables with numerical data

A number of texts provide detailed instructions on the construction of tables. See, for example, Anderson and Poole (1994), Price (1997a, b), and Teitelbaum (1982). Table 17.5 provides an example of a table containing numerical data; it was created using Excel spreadsheet software. Note that the decimal points are lined up vertically and the variables are clearly labelled.

Table 17.5   Scores on three tests of men's and women's attitude towards child-rearing

	Test 1: ACMT (max. 60)*			Test 2: PPS (max. 110)*			Test 3: ATPS (max. 100)*		
	Mean	SD**	%	Mean	SD**	%	Mean	SD**	%
Men	44.3	8.2	73.8	78.3	7.2	71.2	25.4	8.2	25.4
Women	27.5	25.5	45.8	81.4	4.2	74.0	79.9	25.5	79.9
Average	35.9	16.9	59.8	79.9	5.7	72.6	52.7	16.9	52.7

*max. = maximum possible score on test

**SD = standard deviation

Pictures

At times your text, poster, or talk can be enhanced by including a picture such as a cartoon, photograph, or drawing. These may be in the form of hard copies that you paste onto paper or cardboard (for a poster), electronic images that you paste into your word processing document, data presentations (see Chapter 20), or overhead transparency files. Figures 17.4 to 17.6 provide some examples of images that could be included in text. Figure 17.4 was created in a Word file by inserting a clip art image (see Figure 17.4). Figure 17.5 was created in Word using the drawing facility (use DRAWING toolbar, AUTOSHAPES and FILL options for shading). Remember to group your images so that the whole finished graphic stays intact as you position it in your document or repaginate your file. Figure 17.6 was created in Paint Shop Pro by editing a photograph and using EDIT, PASTE SPECIAL to insert it in a Word file.

Figure 17.4 Clip art

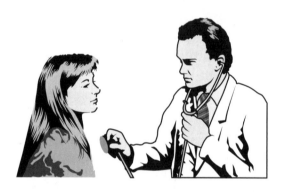

Figure 17.5 Factors influencing health in the elderly

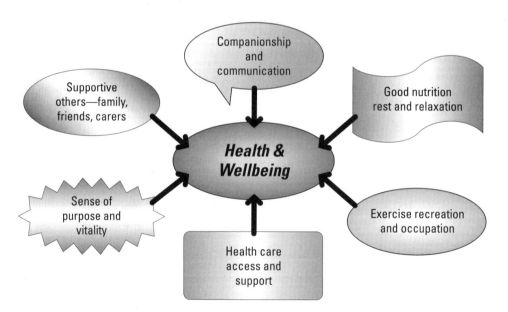

Figure 17.6   Images of health care

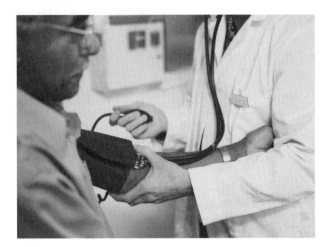

Labelling graphics

Different professions and disciplines have different conventions for using and labelling graphics. You should check with your university's assignment guidelines or ask your lecturers to find out what local expectations you need to follow.

17.2 Numbering and labelling graphics

All graphics, figures, and tables must be numbered. They may be numbered sequentially through the whole work (e.g. Figure 1, Figure 2, etc.) or through each chapter (e.g. Table 1.1, Table 1.2, etc., in Chapter 1, and Table 2.1, Table 2.2, etc., in Chapter 2). Number each type of graphic separately. Each graphic, figure, and table also needs a concise label explaining what is is about. A longer description or discussion of the content of the illustration should occur in the text, but there's no need to duplicate all the information from graphics, tables, and figures in the text. All illustrations must be referred to in the text, to indicate how they relate to your argument.

HANDY HINT

Conclusion

Look at each of the graphics and tables in this chapter and ask yourself the following questions:
• How did the graphic/table add value to the chapter?
• What information can be obtained from this graphic/table?
• What can I learn from this exercise about how to construct a graph, table, or figure?

References

Adler, R. B. & Rodman, G. 2003, *Understanding Human Communication*, 8th edn, Oxford University Press, New York.

Anderson, J. & Poole, M. 2001, *Thesis and Assignment Writing*, 4th edn, John Wiley & Sons, Milton, Qld.

Baker, E., Barrett, M. & Roberts, L. 2002, *Working Communication*, John Wiley & Sons, Milton, Qld.

Hay, I., Bochner, D. & Dungey, C. 2002, *Making the Grade: A Guide to Successful Communication and Study*, Oxford University Press, Melbourne.

Price, C. 1997a, 'How to produce clear tables and figures: Part 1', in G. Allison, *Scientific Writer's Handbook*, Australian Journal of Physiotherapy monograph, Melbourne, pp. 28–35.

Price, C. 1997b, 'How to produce clear tables and figures: Part 2', in G. Allison, *Scientific Writer's Handbook*, Australian Journal of Physiotherapy monograph, Melbourne, pp. 36–45.

Teitelbrum, H. 1982, *How to Write a Thesis: A Guide to the Research Paper*, Monarch Press, New York.

18 | PREPARING POSTERS

Iain Hay and Ann Sefton

KEY TOPICS

→ Reasons for preparing a poster

→ Characteristics of a successful poster

Designing a poster:

→ layout and research

→ elements of a poster

→ number of words

→ guiding the reader

→ Matters of visibility and colour: text and type, colour, figures, and photos

→ Acknowledging sources

Introduction

Posters are a useful way of presenting the results of research and other information to classmates and to scholarly and public audiences. You need a combination of graphic and written skills to ensure your posters achieve their potential to communicate with power and simplicity. Posters can encourage informal discussion, convey vital public health information, and quickly transmit the results of a scientific study. They are an increasingly common and important form of communication at scientific and professional conferences (Sweeney 1984; Hinzmann 1996). At conferences, posters may be on display or presenters may be asked to be present during poster sessions to discuss the material (e.g. research) contained in the poster, or give a short talk (e.g. 5 minutes) on the research to foster discussion or questions.

A poster is commonly a piece of stiff card of dimensions no less than 90 x 60 cm to which materials such as graphs, charts, tables, and photos are affixed, linked together by a small amount of text. There are four key characteristics of a good poster:

- It makes a good first impression. Clever layout and good use of colour help grab the attention of the audience.
- It is coherent and self-contained. A poster cannot rely on additional explanation to make sense.
- It is supported by accurate, appropriately referenced evidence.
- It is as brief as possible.

HANDY HINT

18.1   Transporting posters

Sometimes it is more convenient for transporting a poster to prepare it as a series of 'pages' (e.g. nine A4 laminated pages prepared using PowerPoint), which can be affixed using velcro dots to a poster display board provided by the conference organisers or university staff. (You will need to check if this display option is available.)

Poster layout and text

Good layout is vital to effective graphic communication. Posters do not have to be set up in a linear form, with readers moving from top left to bottom right. A variety of alternatives exist, including cyclical diagrams and spider diagrams. A couple of examples are shown in Figure 18.1. Just as you should prepare an essay plan, it is a good idea to produce sketch diagrams or mock-ups of your poster before you begin the final version. Experiment with different layouts and discuss them with friends and tutors, but whatever design you choose it is essential that the reader has a clear sense of direction through the poster. Numbers, arrows, or headings that reflect well-known procedural sequences (e.g. Introduction, Methods, and Results) may be helpful. Keep each section consistent in style.

Academic and public information posters almost always contain some text. Together with the graphics, the text contributes to the introduction, explanation, and discussion of the work. Keep text to a minimum. Some authors (e.g. Lethbridge 1991) have suggested a maximum word count of 500, and Lethbridge also argued that a poster will be most effective if it uses

HANDY HINT

18.2   Creating posters on computer

Software such as PowerPoint can be used to create professional-looking posters quickly. AUTOLAYOUT functions provide options very suitable for poster construction. The software allows you to insert images and text and apply arrows, numbered boxes, and so on. Once produced electronically, the poster can be printed at an appropriate size (depending on your printer) and possibly enlarged on a photocopier, or it may need to be sent to a commercial printery.

Figure 18.1   Two forms of poster layout

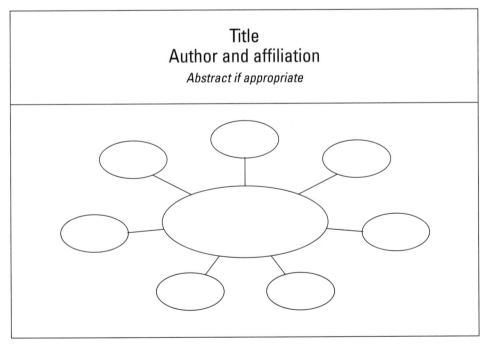

Source: Adapted from Hay & Thomas 1999

only 250–400 words. The text should be in large print and confined to short sections complementing the poster's graphic components, since audiences do not enjoy reading long blocks of text on posters (Welch & Waehler 1996). The text on an academic poster is typically set out in six or seven parts:

1   The *title* (and any *subheadings*) must be succinct. It also helps if the title is memorable and effectively summarises the subject, so that your poster will attract the right audience. Immediately underneath the title present your name and your professional affiliation (or your class/group) and, if appropriate, your contact details (e.g. email address). The title is probably the most important single element of a poster because it influences people's decision over whether to examine the rest of the poster, so think about it carefully.

2   An *abstract* is a short written statement summarising the key points of the poster. This usually appears immediately under the title and your name. Not all posters need an abstract. It is most commonly expected of posters presented at professional conferences.

3   An *introduction* makes clear the aims of the work. Set the scene, explain what is already known (referring to the work of others), and say why your work is worthwhile. If your work has experimental hypotheses, state those in this section.

4   The poster then includes several key sections in which the topic or report is presented. This could include the following sections if the poster is reporting on research:
    > A *materials and methods* section explains the research techniques you used. You should also tell the reader about the study's precision.
    > The *results* are a key part of the poster. Almost every reader will want to see compelling evidence in this section if they are to believe your conclusions. Set out the primary data on which your conclusions are based.
    > A *conclusions* section tells the reader how you interpreted the data. It also refers back to information from the introduction to remind the reader of the data's disciplinary and social significance, and it may set out your plans for future work in the area.
    Alternatively, you may have set out to investigate how a particular service (e.g. mental health practice in your profession) operates. In this case you could include headings like:
    > the goals of mental health care
    > mental health settings and services
    > mental health from the client's perspective
    > resources and resource people.

5   A final section, such as a *conclusion*, *summary* or *reflections* section, sums up the main messages in the poster.

6   *References* to all work cited in the poster should also be set out, usually in the lower right-hand corner.

HANDY HINT ☞ 18.3   Poster layout

Try laying out and rearranging the draft sections of your poster on a table, the floor, or a piece of poster board until you have found a format that is logical and appealing to the eye. If you are using software such as PowerPoint to create your poster, you can do the same thing electronically.

A poster should be accurate and comprehensible even though the text needs to be concise. Do not set out all the details of the project or topic your poster is reporting on, or it could be too crowded, but bear in mind that a good poster does not require further explanation for someone to make sense of it. If anyone is especially interested in the work or issue the poster describes, they can contact you. Furthermore, they could consult some of the literature in the reference list.

Legibility, font, and colour

Everything on a poster should be legible from a distance of about 1.5 metres. Titles and headings should be visible to viewers several metres away, and, to further promote ease of reading, text should employ both upper- and lower-case letters (called 'sentence case'), *not* all capitals, WHICH ARE A LOT MORE DIFFICULT TO READ. Text should be presented in a series of short statements. Do not make the mistake of creating a poster that is simply an essay pasted onto a board.

Suggested font sizes for posters are set out in Table 18.1. Larger size fonts can be used for short headings; smaller fonts for long titles. Twelve point is a common size for typed essays and reports but it is much too small for any text on a poster.

Type is an important aspect of poster design, especially in relation to headings. Where you can, use a typeface that suits the subject material. While the body of the text needs to be clear and simple, extra graphic character and meaning can be added to the poster through the choice of a suitable type (see Table 18.1). For example, **Bookman Old Style** might be appropriate for a poster considering historical aspects of a nation's health-care conditions. By contrast, it might be inappropriate to use Comic Sans MS in a poster about some aspects of HIV/AIDS.

Table 18.1   Fonts for posters

Aspect of font	Description/suggestions		
Typeface	The particular character of the letter forms. There are thousands of typefaces to choose from (e.g. courier, *monotype corsiva*, and **impact**).		
Type weight	The thickness of the letter stroke (e.g., regular and **bold**)		
Type style	This includes *italic*, condensed and extended.		
Type size	Main headings:	96–180 point (27–48.5 mm)	
	Secondary headings:	48–84 point (12.9–25.4 mm)	
	Section headings:	24–36 point (5.9–8.7 mm)	
	Text and captions:	14–18 point (3.2–4.6 mm)	

Colour is a vital part of a poster, either adding to or detracting from the overall impact of the project. It can command attention, bring pleasure, and clarify a point. But you need to use colour with great care. Use a small group of colours to minimise confusion, and give some consideration to matters of colour combination (e.g. blues complement oranges; reds complement greens; yellows complement purples). Colour can add symbolic connotations and feelings to the message of a poster. Table 18.2 summarises some connotations of colour from an Anglo-American perspective.

Take care when choosing combinations of text and background colours to ensure that the text is contrasted with the background and hence is easy to read. For example, black text on a white background is much easier to read than orange on yellow.

A poster on the physiological consequences of heart surgery might effectively employ the colour red to highlight the nature and intensity of the treatment method. By contrast, a

Table 18.2 Some connotations of colour

Colour	Associations
Black	Clear-cut and crisp, death, dignity, doom and gloom, finances
Blue	Calm, climatological, coastal, coolness, rivers, peace, sadness
Brown	Dismal, dreary, earth, pollution, soils
Green	Agriculture, conservation, coolness, envy, freshness, growth, nature, rural, safety, spring, vegetation, wealth
Orange	Autumn, flames, healthiness, sunshine, warmth
Red	Action, blood, danger, financial deficit, fire, hazards, health, heat, Marxism, noise, passion
White	Cleanliness, glory, iciness, purity, snow
Yellow	Beaches, happiness, light-heartedness, sand, sunshine, weakness

Source: Adapted from Sim 1981

Figure 18.2 Poster example

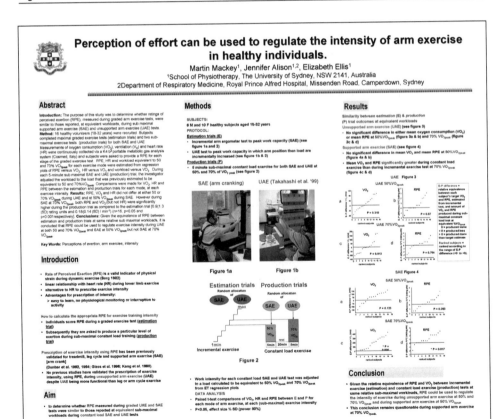

Source: M. Mackey (reproduced with permission)

stark black-and-white poster on AIDS might conjure up physical images of life and death whilst simultaneously raising the spectre of the considerable moral issues that surround the disease. Particular colours are often associated with specific cultures and nations, and they may be useful if you are discussing an issue that is specific to that group; for example, red, yellow, and black are now often associated with the Indigenous populations of Australia. Finally, colour and shading may also be used to add information to particular graphics or to help the reader to interpret otherwise complicated data series.

Using images

Images are another important part of a good poster. The images you use might include a variety of graphics, such as diagrams, cartoons, bar charts, pie diagrams, graphs, and flow charts as well as photographs. Photographs could be used, for example, to compare a healthy mole with a melanoma, and an accompanying diagram could depict some of the abnormal cell growth associated with a melanoma. See Figure 18.2 for an example of a poster.

If you use photographs in your poster, ensure that they are in focus, have sharp contrast, and are sufficiently large to be interpreted from at least 1.5 metres away. A caption should make it clear what a photograph's subject is and, if appropriate, should indicate the degree of magnification used (Singleton 1984). Any images you use in a poster should be of high quality and must be relevant. Do not make the mistake of littering your poster with unnecessary and poor-quality graphs and photographs.

Conclusion

Finally, remember that a poster tells a story or presents an argument, a topic review, or a research report. Make your points clear and the poster entertaining.

References

Briscoe, M. H. 1996, *Preparing Scientific Illustrations: A Guide to Better Posters, Presentations, and Publications*, 2nd edn, Springer, New York.

Gosling, P. J. 1999, *Scientist's Guide to Poster Presentations*, Kluwer Academic, New York.

Hay, I. & Thomas, S. 1999, 'Making sense with posters in biological science education', *Journal of Biological Education*, vol. 33, no. 4, pp. 209–14.

Hinzmann, C. 1996, 'BSN students present research findings on complex health problems in poster session format', *Journal of Nursing Education*, vol. 35, no. 4, pp. 177–8.

Lethbridge, R. 1991, *Techniques for Successful Seminars and Poster Presentations*, Longman Cheshire, Melbourne.

Sim, R. 1981, *Lettering for Signs, Projects, Posters, Displays*, 2nd edn, Learning Publications, Balgowlah, Australia.

Singleton, A. 1984, *Poster Sessions: A Guide to Their Use at Meetings and Conferences—For Presenters and Organisers*, Elsevier, Oxford.

Sweeney, S. S. 1984, 'Poster sessions for undergraduate students: A useful tool for learning and communicating nursing research', *Western Journal of Nursing Research*, vol. 6, no. 1, pp. 135–8.

Welch, A. A. & Waehler, C. A. 1996, 'Preferences about APA poster presentations', *Teaching of Psychology*, vol. 23, no. 1, pp. 42–4.

Further reading

'Scientific posters' <http://miu.med.unsw.edu.au/sci_posters.htm> accessed 17 March 2004.

19 | GIVING TALKS IN CLASS

Annette Street, Iain Hay, and Ann Sefton

KEY TOPICS

→ Reasons to give talks in class

→ Different styles of talks

→ Principles for giving effective talks

→ Introducing, discussing, and concluding

→ Maintaining audience attention

→ Using AV to enhance a presentation

Introduction

Well-developed skills in oral presentation are needed for case presentations, educational sessions in the workplace, and presentations of work at conferences and seminars. One goal of health and social science education therefore is to produce articulate graduates who are skilled in oral presentation. You will undoubtedly be asked to give talks in class. You need to do this confidently and effectively.

Reasons to give talks in class

Addressing an audience can be intimidating even for experienced public speakers. It is a skill that can be developed with time and effort (Burns & Joyce 1997). Those who appear to speak effortlessly in public are always well prepared (Bly 2003). They understand their topic and the restrictions on what can be presented in the time available, and they have the capacity to pepper their talk with humour, stories, images, statistics, and enough repetition to make their points effectively (Ayres & Ayres 2003); these are skills you can develop. They have also developed skills in the process of presenting talks, including the ability to use audiovisual (AV) aids effectively and to present in a relaxed, seemingly effortless manner (without distracting fidgeting, mumbling, shuffling of papers, or fumbling with AV equipment). The advice given here on the use of common AV aids is also relevant to the use of PowerPoint presentations and other forms of data projection, as detailed in Chapter 20.

While you are a student, you will be asked to give talks in class to help you learn to organise and present your ideas logically and clearly. You are preparing for a career in one of the health and social science professions, in all of which oral presentation skills are an important professional proficiency. You will need to learn how to adapt your material to the purpose of the talk, the level of formality, the likely audience, the venue, and the allocated time (Schmoll 2002).

Talks in class develop a range of skills. You may be required to investigate evidence on a topic and then to present it in class to inform and educate your fellow students. Your task might be to advocate a particular solution to a health-related problem on the basis of the relevant literature. Debating skills will help you to prepare and present an argument and persuade your audience to adopt your point of view. Another task might be to respond to the presentations of others in a clear and constructive manner. Similar skills are needed for case presentations, which are central to many disciplines.

Different styles of talk

Common forms of class talks require different styles of presentation, and the style of presentation will govern how a talk is developed and the way the material is presented (see Table 19.1).

Table 19.1 Forms of presentation

Style of presentation	Key focus
Tutorial	Students may be asked to present a topic they have prepared. Transmission of information is usually one-way, although questions may be encouraged.
Project report	Students who have worked on a project inform others of their findings. Sometimes a group coordinates the presentation, with each member of the group taking a section.
Case presentation	Students present the case of a patient or client, to encourage discussion of possible diagnoses, therapies, medications, parameters, or prognoses.
Class discussion	A student leads a discussion of a designated topic. The intention is not primarily to transmit information but to evaluate it from a range of perspectives.
Debate	A proposition is set. Each speaker is required to argue for or against it, aiming to persuade the audience.
Oral defence (or viva)	Students are required to summarise the key arguments, findings, and conclusions of their thesis or essay and to answer questions from an informed audience in order to demonstrate their understanding.

Speaking to an audience you know well

Different audiences bring different challenges. If you know members of the audience, you will probably have a clear idea of their level of knowledge and the expectations they bring with them. In giving a talk to your class, one advantage is that you already know something about your audience. But sometimes your fellow students or colleagues can be difficult to address. They may make assumptions about you and your abilities, based on their prior knowledge of you. Also, it can be difficult or intimidating to speak in front of people you know well and will continue to see in the future. Nevertheless, this will be a common task after you graduate, as part of your professional practice. It is important to learn to address colleagues and fellow students with the same degree of confidence and authority that you would have with an unknown audience. In class presentations it is often better to be somewhat formal, as you want to present in such a way that your audience takes you seriously, respecting your information and analysis.

When preparing a talk for people you know already, think about which aspects will be of most interest to them. How can you capture their attention? Perhaps start by focusing on new, interesting ideas rather than rehashing all the known points, although you may need to orient them to the issues you will discuss. Starting with lists of data will bore your audience. Instead, consider using a story or an example to set complex information in context. This will help your audience to understand the important ideas related to the topic.

Your in-class audience will include not only your classmates but also one or more teachers. They will typically be making judgments based on your presentation of new knowledge. They will evaluate whether your material is based on good evidence, whether your arguments are well-structured and compelling, and whether your conclusions make sense. They will also assess your understanding and the breadth and depth of your reading by the sophistication of your arguments, your synthesis of the material, and the way you handle questions. You may have received a marking sheet in advance or otherwise know how marks will be awarded (e.g. for presentation, content, audience participation, etc.); this will help you plan and present a good talk.

You must prepare thoroughly if you want to look and feel confident. Remember that speech is structured differently from written language, so you need to take care to write in the way you would speak. Practise your talk aloud. Speak slowly, as you will speed up if you are nervous. Think about how you stand and any mannerisms you might have. These can be more obvious in class than when you are behind a lectern. Holding onto your notes or the lectern can help you avoid irritating and distracting hand movements or shuffling feet. As classrooms often don't provide lecterns, you should develop and practise using a strategy for managing all your overheads and notes (e.g. use a table for the used and unused overheads and hold your notes on cards in your hands). You could ask a friend or co-presenter to change the overhead transparencies for you so that you can concentrate on the talk and on engaging the audience. Don't put things on a low table or chair as your audience will see a lot of the top of your head and not your face.

Use short, concise sentences and practise your timing. If you expect your audience to react at certain points by laughing at an anecdote or reading an overhead, leave time for this. As you become more familiar with your talk you may decide not to read it. You can reduce your notes to the introductory sentences, prompts, and key points, keeping the full script as a fall-back. If you choose to do this, highlight the key points in your text so that you can reorient yourself if you decide to break from the script and elaborate on a point. Or make up some prompt cards that list each main point and prompts. You are more likely to remain calm in class and speak well if you are serious about careful preparation.

Practising the presentation also means practising the operation and timing of your AV aids. How long do they take to set up? Do you need a particular room arrangement? Do you know how to operate the equipment? One of the first things to do when preparing for your talk is to establish which AV aids will be available. You may need to book them ahead of time. You will also need to know the size of the room or hall, so that you can prepare visual aids that can be read easily from the back row. The most reliable, readily available, and simple visual support for your presentation is still an overhead projector. You can summarise your main points and provide graphs, flowcharts, or raw data on overhead transparencies to support your argument.

19.1   Preparing for class talks

* Consider what class members know and what they don't know.
* Prepare an interesting start.
* Check your argument and evidence.
* Write out your script in full, remembering to use language that you would naturally use in speech.
* Break it down to key points and prompts.
* Practice aloud and standing.
* Be somewhat formal; you should give the talk as if the class were strangers. (You may want to be more relaxed and less formal when it comes to question time or promoting discussion.)

HANDY HINT

Introducing, discussing, and concluding

The start and finish of presentations are important. During the introduction you set out the framework of your presentation. Your audience needs to be clear on what to expect. At the end you summarise the key points and emphasise the main message. You present your key arguments and discuss their implications in the body of the presentation.

Introduction

To give a clear and effective introduction, you should do the following:
* Introduce the topic! Do this in an interesting manner, without rushing. Before you start speaking take a deep breath, establish good eye contact, and smile.
* State the aim of the talk, so that the listeners will be clear about your approach to the topic and what you intend to achieve.
* Define the scope, depth, and limits of the presentation, so that the audience will know what to expect.
* Provide an outline of the key points; this will make it easier for the audience to follow your argument.

You will assert more authority in class if you are tidily dressed and well organised. Maintain a good posture and establish eye contact by looking around the room at everyone, particularly at the outset. Don't just focus on your friends or your notes. You need to impress on your classmates and teachers that you are here to present your ideas and analysis in an engaging way. Start with an interesting fact, anecdote, story, or visual. Avoid jokes, as the audience may get the message that you do not expect them to pay serious attention to you.

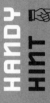

HANDY HINT ☞ 19.2   Maintaining audience attention

- Make an attention-grabbing start.
- Pose thought-provoking questions that keep the audience involved.
- Stay in control of your material.
- Adhere to your outline.
- Pace the presentation and do not try to cover too much.
- Use simple, effective visual aids.
- Maintain eye contact and don't fidget.

Table 19.2   Advantages and disadvantages of various visual aids

Type	Advantages	Disadvantages
Whiteboard	• Reinforces main points • Allows for use of colour • Good for building up a series of connected ideas • Easy to organise, and can be used outdoors	• Not good for large and/or complicated diagrams • Not useful for large audiences • You usually have to turn your back to the audience • Requires clear handwriting
Flipchart or paper pad stand	• Inexpensive and easily transported • Important material can be prepared in advance • Prompts can be pencilled in beforehand	• Suitable only for small groups • You usually have to turn your back to the audience • Needs a stable easel for support • Requires clear handwriting
Prepared poster	• Provides a brief striking message • Can include complex colour and design elements	• Can be large and awkward to carry • Can be costly to design well
Overhead transparency projector (OHP)	• Images can be seen by everyone • Good for pre-prepared material using colours or diagrams • Can be prepared from computer-generated slides • No need to turn away from audience • Can use overlays • Can be masked so you can reveal information gradually • Can be stored and reused	• Needs a power source • Needs to be correctly aligned • Projector bulbs can fail without warning • Material can be too small to be read • Transparencies can be awkward to manage
Slides	• Images are of better quality than with OHP • Better at displaying pictures and photographs than OHP • Can be stored and reused	• Projector needs a power source and a darkened room • Needs preparation of slide alignment, projector focus, etc. • Expensive to produce

Table 19.2 Advantages and disadvantages of various visual aids (continued)

Type	Advantages	Disadvantages
Computer-generated visual with data projector	• Relatively easy to combine text, graphics, audio and video • Can generate a sophisticated product relatively cheaply	• Needs a power source • Needs a computer and projector • Technical difficulties in usage are common
Real object	• May be readily available and convenient to display • Audience can see how object works and looks, and it can be used	• May not be suitable for large groups • Potential for damage to object • Not appropriate for large objects
Model	• Works well for large objects • Gives audience sense of scale and of relationships between elements of the object	• May not be to scale • Detail may not be seen by audience • Potential for damage to model • Potentially costly to produce

Source: Derived from Baker et al. 2002

Results

In some talks you will be presenting your own (or your group's) findings from practical classes, fieldwork, or research projects. Make your main points clearly, and provide concise evidence or examples. If you are presenting as a member of a team, plan beforehand the sequence and scope of each person's contribution, and practise your timing as a group, to ensure that you all get your fair share of the presentation time.

Use your AV material to signal key points, identify new topics, show the structure (e.g. outline of the talk), and present the summary and conclusions. You can also prepare additional material (e.g. extra transparencies) to answer anticipated questions. Prepare your visual aids to have some commonality and continuity for greatest impact. Table 19.2 (based on Baker et al. 2002) provides an overview of the advantages and disadvantages of different forms of visual communication.

Discussion

The body of the talk needs to be well structured into a logical argument supported by strong evidence. Keep in mind that the the best public speakers try to organise their material into a few main arguments, with an overarching take-home message. Design an outline (an overhead, handout, or PowerPoint presentation) to show your key points and any sub-themes. Use it to orient your audience throughout the talk. If appropriate, provide a personal example related to the topic, or explain how you have thought about these ideas.

When possible, provide support for the points you are making in the form of a diagram, chart, or table. If you don't have diagrams, consider supporting some points with quotations. But don't overload any visual with too much text, and don't read exactly what your audience can read on the screen. If you want to tell a story or read a quote, put just the key points on your visual.

Keep the presentation simple. Keep the focus on you. Don't try to use flashy visual effects or other strategies that may backfire or distract the audience from your message. If you have presented your own class or research findings, you may introduce briefly one or two examples of the findings of others, indicating how they corroborate or conflict with your results.

Conclusion

The conclusion is where you tell the audience what you want them to remember. It will help if you:

- use your AV or handout outline to remind your audience of the key points and signal that you want to make concluding remarks
- 'sell' your take-home message and reinforce it with an arresting image or compelling statistic.
- tie in your take-home message with your introduction.

Finish your presentation by thanking your audience for listening. A simple 'Thank you' is much more effective and professional than the lame 'Well, I guess that's about it …', which is often uttered!

Question time

You are usually expected to answer questions about your talk. Most people feel anxious about this. Don't rush to answer. Stop briefly and consider what the question means. If you are not sure, repeat or paraphrase the question in your own words and check if that was what the questioner wanted to know. Repeat questions aloud if some people in the audience cannot hear them. Often people ask long questions with multiple parts. Break up long questions into parts and answer each part. You may need to jot down the separate parts on your notes. If a question is off the topic of your presentation, then say so (politely) and move on to the next question. If you don't know the answer to a question, say so; you might also consider asking members of the audience if they can shed any light on the problem. If the question is obviously of interest to the questioner only, suggest that they talk to you about it after the presentation.

When you answer a question, look occasionally at the questioner but direct your answer to the whole group. Don't allow one questioner to dominate question time. If possible, use the final question to reacquaint your audience with your take-home message.

Every health or social science student needs to learn how to plan and deliver an effective talk (Turner 2002). Almost everyone is nervous about public speaking, but you can become a good speaker if you plan the content and presentation carefully. Case Study 19.1 reveals how a lack of preparation can jeopardise a presentation.

19.1

CASE STUDY

Poor preparation for presentation

A colleague presented some of his work in a hospital meeting. He had prepared his material on prompt cards with key points and a series of overheads of statistical results. But he hadn't practised standing and talking with his prompt cards or managing the overheads on the overhead projector. The lighting was poor, making it hard for him to read his cards without holding his arm out. This meant he could not make eye contact with his audience. He also dropped his overheads when he tried to change them while still holding his prompt card. He became nervous and apologetic and some people walked out. What would you have done if you had been in this situation?

References

Ayres, J. & Ayres, T. A. 2003, 'Using images to enhance the impact of visualization', *Communication Reports*, vol. 16, no. 1, pp. 47–55.

Baker, E., Barrett, M. & Roberts, L. 2002, *Working Communication*, John Wiley & Sons, Milton, Qld.

Bly, R. W. 2003, 'Give memorable presentations', *Chemical Engineering Progress*, vol. 99, no. 1, pp. 84–7.

Burns, A. & Joyce, H. 1997, *Focus on Speaking*, National Centre for English Language Teaching and Research, North Ryde, NSW, Australia.

Schmoll, B. J. 2002, 'Writing, speaking, and communication skills for health professionals', *Physical Therapy*, vol. 82, no. 5, pp. 524–5.

Turner, J. 2002, *How to Study: A Short Introduction*, Sage Publications, London.

20 | POWERPOINT PRESENTATIONS

Charles Higgs and Joy Higgs

KEY TOPICS

→ Why use PowerPoint presentations?

→ When should they be used?

→ How to prepare your files

→ Planning your presentation

→ Using PowerPoint

Introduction

Increasingly, students are using computer-based presentations in classroom presentations and at conferences. To make such a presentation, you need to design a file containing a series of electronic slides, using software such as PowerPoint, then load this file onto a computer and connect a data projector to project the file onto a screen. (Throughout this chapter we refer to PowerPoint, but the principles and strategies would be similar for most presentation software.) Electronic presentations enhance talks in classes and conferences because they are more flexible and feature-rich than overhead projector transparencies. They are rapidly becoming the standard at conferences. In classes, there are times when other media, such as overhead projectors and whiteboards, are preferable, for example if the discussion is interactive or evolving and

184

the presenter/facilitator does not want to restrict or cannot predict the desired content or sequence of the slides. Use the presentation medium that is applicable to the situation.

What makes a good PowerPoint presentation?

Think about any PowerPoint presentations you have seen. What did you like or not like about these presentations? The following factors are important:

* *Timing.* Make sure your talk and your slides match in terms of the numbers of slides and key points. Check that your technology (e.g. complex animation) does not waste time or detract from your talk.
* *Suitability* for the audience. Is your presentation too simplistic, complex, irrelevant, or repetitive?
* *Readability.* If you use complex slides (e.g. graphs and tables), make sure that people have time to read them. Sometimes it might be a good idea to prepare a handout containing these slides. Slides that contain too much information are hard to read (e.g. because the font is too small).
* *Entertainment.* As well as presenting information, your talk should engage your audience. Graphics (see Chapter 17) can help you keep your audience's attention.

Planning your PowerPoint presentation

The first stage in designing a PowerPoint presentation is planning your accompanying talk. Chapters 19 and 21 will help you with that task. There are five steps to preparing the actual presentation.

1. Identify your objective

The first step in planning a presentation is to decide what you want to achieve and what you want your audience to get out of the presentation. Is your presentation about a health-care technique you want to inform your audience about, are you trying to 'sell' an idea, or are you simply trying to present information in a clear and logical manner?

2. Consider your audience

'What's in it for me?' is the subconscious question asked by your audience. Putting yourself in their shoes will help you to anticipate any questions and issues that might arise, and, more importantly, it will allow you to plan your presentation around their needs. Some of the aspects you should consider are the audience's values, beliefs, needs, interests, and background knowledge.

You need to engage with your audience. Using PowerPoint should enhance your talk. It should be interesting and informative without taking over from what you have to say or distracting your audience. You can engage your audience through the use of appropriate images, clip art, movie sound bites, etc. Remember that you can blank the presentation (press the key B) if you want the audience to concentrate on your talk rather than the screen (press the key B again to resume the presentation).

3. Plan your content and graphics

It's a good idea to write down the key points you want to include in your PowerPoint presentation and plan the graphics you want to include in your talk. Graphics can include graphs (prepared using Excel or another spreadsheet program), tables (e.g. Word or Excel tables), pictures (e.g. scanned or digital photographs), and images (e.g. clip art images). You may use a graphics program (e.g. Paint Shop Pro or PhotoShop) to prepare and edit the pictures, or use the drawing features built into PowerPoint.

4. Visit the venue

If possible you should visit the venue where you are going to give your presentation. You should consider the following things:

- What equipment is there (and how do I use it)?
- What type of computer is provided?
- Is the software of the same type and version as I used to create my presentation?
- Do I need to bring my presentation on floppy disc, on CD, or in some other form? (A CD is commonly needed for presentations with photos and detailed graphics, as most floppy disks cannot hold such large files.)
- Will I have technical support?
- How will the audience be seated and where will I be positioned in relation to the audience?
- Do I know how to use the lecture theatre controls for data projection, lighting, and the microphone?

5. Practise your timing

When you are practising your presentation with PowerPoint, remember to monitor your timing. As a rule of thumb, use one slide for approximately 5–6 minutes of your talk. You can use SLIDE SHOW/REHEARSE TIMING to determine how long your slide show will take. If you want an unbiased review of your presentation, deliver it to your family or classmates.

Creating a simple PowerPoint presentation

There are a number of free tutorials available on the Internet on using PowerPoint (see the list at the end of this chapter). Some of these tutorials are extremely useful and cover far more features than we can cover in the space of this chapter. Use your favourite search engine (Google is a good choice) and use 'powerpoint+tutorials' in your search.

The following steps will guide you through the creation of a simple PowerPoint presentation. Note that the steps described relate to PowerPoint 2002, but the process is similar in other versions of PowerPoint. Later in this chapter we look at aspects of how to create a more complex presentation.

HANDY HINT

20.1 Alternatives

There is often more than one way to do a task and you should choose the technique that suits your computer style. For example, adding a new slide can be achieved using any of the following options:

- INSERT, NEW SLIDE
- Ctrl-M
- the 'New Slide' symbol

1. Opening a file

Open PowerPoint on your computer and choose FILE, NEW. Choose VIEW, NORMAL. Note that the screen typically has three sections (depending upon your PowerPoint version and configuration). The left column shows a series of slide icons. The central section is the working area for the current slide. The right section contains common tasks associated with the action you are currently undertaking (e.g. if you are adding new slides the right section displays the available slide layouts).

2. Choosing a template

PowerPoint has a number of inbuilt templates (background images and associated text formats) that you can choose for your presentation. You can choose a template by selecting FORMAT, SLIDE DESIGN (or clicking on the Design icon) and choosing your preferred template. An example of a template is shown in Figure 20.1. You may wish to create your own

Figure 20.1 Slide template and dot point layout

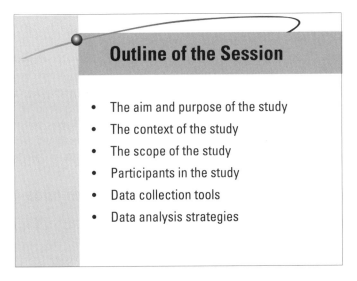

Figure 20.2 Picture as background

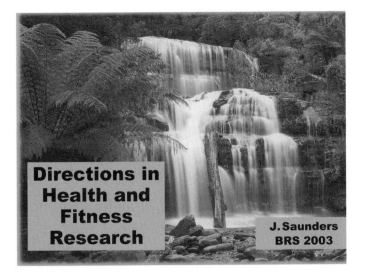

slide background design. Select FORMAT, BACKGROUND and click on the colour bar to choose a colour or fill effect, or add a picture to use as your background (see Figure 20.2). For advanced files, experiment with the use of master slides and layers of graphics on your slides.

HANDY HINT ☞ 20.2 Projecting in large lecture theatres

In conference presentations it is often desirable to avoid having a dark background with light text, which can be difficult to read in large lecture theatres.

3. Adding slides and text

PowerPoint has a number of inbuilt slide formats, such as title slides, table slides, and list slides (see Figure 20.1). Open a new slide by clicking on INSERT, NEW SLIDE and choose your desired format. Type directly onto the slide or cut your prepared Word text and paste it onto your slide. Save your file frequently, so that you do not lose your work.

Remember that the whole point of using data projection is to provide a clear, readable visual image to complement your talk. In terms of text lines, we suggest you follow the 7x7 rule; that is, use a maximum of seven words per line and seven lines per slide. Use text that is clear and easy to read: avoid using ALL CAPITALS, use a minimum font size of 18, and use a simple font, such as Arial or Helvetica.

HANDY HINT ☞ 20.3 Testing the legibility of slides

Print out one slide from your presentation and lay it on the ground. Take two steps back. If you can still read the slide comfortably, it should be fine with the data projector. Try it out with a data projector and then compare the results. You may have to take three paces instead of two; develop your own rule of thumb from this technique.

4. Adding notes for your talk

As an option, you can insert notes for your talk in the notes section underneath the slide you are working on. You can print out the notes pages to refer to during your talk, by choosing FILE, PRINT, PRINT WHAT, NOTES PAGE. (Note: Don't use the print icon.)

5. Adding clip art

You can add clip art to your presentation by choosing INSERT, PICTURE, CLIP ART. PowerPoint comes with a large selection of built-in clip art.

6. Adding photos, tables, and graphs

On some slides you may want to insert a picture. To do this, open your picture file in a graphics package, copy the image to the clipboard, and then select EDIT, PASTE SPECIAL to put this image on the slide (see Figure 20.3). You can then open a text box to add text. Choose INSERT, TEXTBOX.

Figure 20.3   Slide with photograph

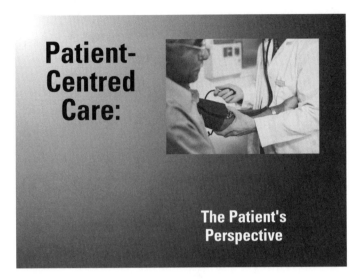

You can also add a flowchart (Figure 20.4), graph (Figure 20.5), or data table from Excel by copying this graphic and using EDIT, PASTE SPECIAL to add it to PowerPoint. This allows you to double click on the graphic to change it as desired (e.g. change colours, size, and font).

Figure 20.4   Slide with flowchart

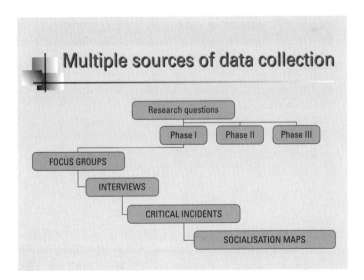

Tables come in different formats. Look at Figure 20.6 (this was Table 17.4 from Chapter 17). You will notice that in importing this table into PowerPoint we have decreased the number of words, used a clearer, bolded font, and adjusted the column width for maximum clarity and readability.

Figure 20.5   Slide with graph

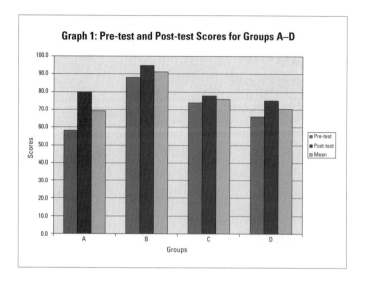

Figure 20.6   Slide with table

Table 1: Theories of benchmarking

Theory	Content	Reference
Best current national practice	• 3 key indicators • Top national hospital	Frederickson 1999
Best international model	• 10 key indicators measured • Top scoring unit/indicator	Schmidt & Abrendt 2001
Achievable growth target	• Own unit as benchmark • Achievable growth	Wu & Fenwick 2000
Ideal position model	• Design ideal model • 6 key parameters	Trendle 2000

Some photos will require editing before you insert them into your PowerPoint presentation. You might need to lighten or darken a photo, change its colours, crop (trim) it, resize it, or add text (for example, by inserting a text box or adding word art). Figure 20.7 illustrates some of the possibilities. Note that if the size of the graphics file is very large, this will increase the overall size of your PowerPoint file, which may become to large to fit on a disk or too slow to load. Burning the file onto a CD could address the first of these problems. Be aware that graphics such as photos can be saved in a number of formats, including JPG, TIF, BMP, and GIF. If the image is a photo or a colour scan of an image, it will probably

Figure 20.7 Editing a photograph

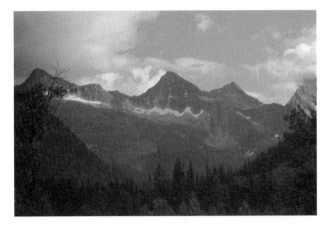

Original

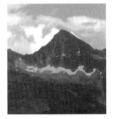

Cropped

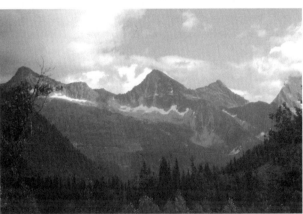

Improved exposure

be best to save and insert it as a JPG file. If the image is clip art or a line drawing that you have scanned, it will usually be best to save it as a GIF image before importing it into your PowerPoint presentation.

7. Inserting hyperlinks

There are three main uses for hyperlinks. You can hyperlink:

- to an external file, website, PDF file, movie, etc. This is useful when you need a link to an active website (remember that you will need a LAN connection or a modem).
- to another presentation. This is useful if you have landscape and portrait presentations and want to move between them.
- to other pages within this presentation. Use this if you have a non-linear presentation and you want to include a menu at the beginning of the presentation and a 'go to menu' link on each page. PowerPoint also has built-in menu buttons (to add select SLIDESHOW, ACTION BUTTONS) that can be loaded onto the master slide and used to navigate through the show.

You can hyperlink to a website, PDF file, etc., from an object like a piece of text, an image, clip art, etc., by selecting the object and choosing INSERT, HYPERLINK, and then selecting the name of the external file, website, PDF file, movie, etc.

8. Editing your presentation

When you have completed all of your slides, save your file. Then it is time to check your presentation. Choose VIEW, SLIDE SORTER and check the sequence of your slides. You can select a slide and drag it to a new position. At the same time, look at the slide formats and identify slides that are not consistent. For example, you may have decided to use Arial font but the text you pasted from Word was in Times New Roman. Fix this using FORMAT, FONT. To spell-check your work, click on TOOLS, LANGUAGE and choose ENGLISH, AUSTRALIAN, then click on TOOLS, SPELLING and follow the prompts. Also read your work, because the spell-checker does not detect all errors (such as 'where' instead of 'were'). Check and fix any errors in text alignment.

To animate or not?

You can make your presentation more visually exciting by adding animation. Animation can be in the form of slide transition (how slides change from one to another) or in the form of individual features within a slide (e.g. bullets or graphics such as boxes and arrows that appear one by one when you click the mouse or after a set time lapse).

HANDY HINT ☞ **20.4 Using animation wisely**

Animation can enliven a presentation but should be used to add value to the presentation, rather than just because the features are available. You do not want to spoil your presentation by emphasising gimmicks rather than your message. Remember the objective of your presentation, your time-frame, and your audience when deciding what animation to use.

Slide transition

Rather than just having one slide disappear and another appear as you move though your presentation, you can use slide transitions to make the presentation more visually stimulating. For example, you can make one slide 'dissolve' into the next, or have the next slide appear via a 'checkerboard' effect. To add a transition select SLIDE SHOW, SLIDE TRANSITION.

Slide animation

It can be an advantage to control how images and text appear on the screen. For example, you may want your bulleted text to appear one line at a time. To achieve this you need to animate the text. Select SLIDE SHOW, CUSTOM ANIMATION and apply the animation to the bulleted text. You can create some powerful effects by animating text and images in your presentation.

Advanced animation

You can apply transitions and other animation elements to more than one slide at a time. If you go into VIEW, SLIDE SORTER, you can select multiple slides by either holding down the SHIFT key and clicking on the first and last slides you want to select, or holding down the CTRL key and clicking on the required slides. Then apply the transition or animation to the selected group.

Practising your presentation

Always practise your presentation and talk using a computer and data projector, preferably in the room in which you will present. This will help you to see how the format, template, and font appear when projected.

Familiarise yourself with PowerPoint's mouse and key commands, so that you can move to previous or later slides. For example, to go back one slide, you can press PAGE UP without revealing the menu, or, if you are in 'show' mode, you can type the number of the slide then hit ENTER to go straight to that screen. This is particularly useful if you have a large show for multiple speakers. Remember to make a note of the slide number at which each speaker starts.

There will be times when you want to stop your presentation and talk to your audience without them being distracted by what is on the screen. Press the letter 'B' to blank out the screen and press 'B' again when you want to restart. If you are using your own computer in a presentation, make sure the screen saver is disabled. It can be embarrassing to be halfway through a presentation and see the screen saver start up!

Print out your notes and handouts. PowerPoint allows you to print out full-page slides, handouts (e.g. six slides to a page), or notes pages containing a slide and any notes you added. These will be valuable when you are practising and presenting your talk.

During your practice sessions, time your presentation and decide whether your talk needs to be extended or shortened. If possible, ask a friend or colleague to listen to your practice presentation and use the feedback to improve your slides or delivery.

Conclusion

An over-arching principle is that your PowerPoint slides and data projections should enhance your talk. With this advice in mind, explore the possibilities that this software provides. Remember, as you do so, that different disciplines (e.g. physiology, public health, occupational therapy) and different professional conferences have their own traditions and expectations in relation to the style of presentation material. It's a good idea to investigate these expectations before preparing a presentation.

Further reading

'PowerPoint class' <http://www2.umist.ac.uk/isd/lwt/apt/ppclass/index.shtml> accessed 24 May 2004.
'PowerPoint 2000 basics tutorial' <http://www.iupui.edu/~webtrain/tutorials/powerpoint2000_basics.html> accessed 24 May 2004.

21

PRESENTING TALKS AT CONFERENCES

Annette Street and Iain Hay

KEY TOPICS

→ Reasons for speaking at a conference

→ Characteristics of an effective presentation

→ Strategies for preparation and presentation

→ Using visual aids

→ Managing questions

Introduction

Speaking at a conference is a vital way of summarising your work for others, positioning yourself as a person working in a particular field, and receiving feedback on your work from colleagues. Although your professional education will give you experience at speaking in class to fellow students (see Chapter 19), it is important to also be able to present your work effectively to professional peers and to respond confidently to their questions and comments. During your professional education, you may have an opportunity to make a presentation (for instance of your honours research) at a conference or seminar at your university or at a professional conference. Or this might be an adventure waiting for you after you enter the workforce.

Speaking at conferences

Knowledge and practice in the health and social sciences are changing at a rapid rate. It is imperative that as members of these professions we keep up to date with the work of our peers and share the results of our practice and research. A conference or professional seminar is one of the best places to hear about cutting-edge advances in your field and to present your ideas. It can be daunting to stand up and talk about your work to an audience of strangers (see Gruhn 2001), but public speaking in various forms is part of the role of professionals. Educating others about our work and ideas is an essential component of our professional responsibility to develop our disciplines (see Schmoll 2002). Likewise, keeping abreast in your field, networking with others, and using feedback constructively are vital to professional development. These skills are valued highly in all the health professions and are best learned early.

Your research supervisor may suggest that you present your work at a particular conference. Conferences are expensive and time-consuming to attend. Do your homework, so that you are not disappointed in your choice. Before you make a decision to attend and to present your work, find out as much as you can about the conference and the likely audience for your work. You may decide to prepare and present a poster (see Chapter 18) or present a paper. Many conferences now encourage students to present their work; some conferences even have a student prize. Some professional associations have student sub-groups that conduct local or national student conferences. If it is your first presentation, you should look out for a conference that has a student focus or encourages practitioners or novice researchers to attend and present. You will then probably find a supportive environment and receive helpful feedback. It will also enable you to meet others with similar interests and establish networks with current and future leaders in your specialty.

Many conferences focus on a major theme, but they invariably have a variety of sub-themes and/or discipline groups, to allow people with shared interests to connect with each other. Professional conferences and scientific meetings commonly feature keynote papers or symposia as well as many short papers or posters reporting technical findings and practice advances, presented in concurrent sessions. Larger scientific meetings can have a huge number of papers, workshops, poster displays, showcases of technical equipment, and discipline-specific meetings happening concurrently, and the audience at your session could be small. Some conferences have longer discursive papers, with more time allocated for discussion.

Your winning abstract

The selection of presentations for conferences commonly occurs via a competitive, peer-reviewed process. Once you have decided which conference you want to attend, the next task is to write a winning abstract so that you are given the opportunity to deliver an oral presentation or present a poster. This requires you to clarify the main arguments and/or research findings you will present, and the mode of delivery of your presentation. Read any requirements for abstracts *carefully*. Your abstract should be matched by an arresting presentation title that reflects the conference theme. You can be imaginative with your presentation titles, but you should not promise more than the final presentation will deliver.

Your abstract should provide a short précis of all the key elements in your paper or poster. Writing a good abstract is essential on three counts. First, the abstract may determine whether your paper is accepted for the conference. It can also influence whether you are asked to deliver a long paper, a short paper, or a poster. Second, potential members of the audience may base their decision on whether or not to come to your presentation entirely on the impressions conveyed by your abstract. Third, abstracts of accepted papers are often reproduced in a book of abstracts that is published or distributed to colleagues interested in your work. Make sure that your abstract covers the main points of your message and that your talk can deliver what you promise. Note that it is commonly bad practice to submit an abstract before your results and conclusions are available. The exception to this is if the abstract is required many months before the conference and you are confident that your work will be finished well before the conference date. Remember that withdrawal of an abstract reflects poorly on the writer.

HANDY HINT ☞ **21.1 Getting started preparing a talk**

- Do your homework on the conference.
- Develop a catchy title for your paper.
- Write a winning abstract.
- Research your target audience.
- Consider the amount of time you have been allocated and what you can cover in that time.
- Examine the content of papers grouped with yours.
- Check out the venue and audio-visual arrangements.

Preliminary preparation

Your abstract is so good that your paper has been accepted for a conference. What happens next? The first rule is that you can never be too prepared. No matter how experienced you are, good preparation is typically needed for an excellent presentation (Tyler et al. 1999). Start planning early. Break down the preparation process into manageable steps and begin work on one or more steps as soon as you receive confirmation of your acceptance as a speaker from the conference organisers. You will need to take into consideration the following factors.

(a) The target audience

Think carefully about the characteristics of your potential audience. What will these people want to know about your work? Your estimation of their level of knowledge will influence the way you develop your paper. Unlike a classroom presentation, in which the audience probably shares your knowledge base, at a conference you may find that the people who attend your presentation have many different professional interests and levels of knowledge. You can deliberately narrow your audience by adding a subtitle such as 'Implications for speech pathology', which should encourage specialists in your area of expertise to attend (and may discourage others).

(b) The amount of time you have been allocated

Conferences have different lengths of time available for presentations. Find out if the time allocated to you allows for questions from the audience or whether these are to be handled in a follow-up session at the end of a series of papers. Managing time is a crucial skill. Audiences appreciate a well-timed presentation, especially if they want to move to attend another session after yours. It is also embarrassing and frustrating if you have to be stopped talking before you have concluded or if people stand up and leave the room before you have finished because you have taken too long.

(c) The content of papers grouped with yours

Conference organisers usually try to create themes in concurrent sessions and group together papers that address similar topics or use similar methods. Being aware of the papers grouped with yours can assist you in the selection of material to be included, emphasised, or ignored. A paper exploring women's experiences of breast cancer could be grouped by organisers with papers on body image or on breast cancer treatments. The grouping decisions will affect the audience that attends the series of papers in the session and will alert you to their probable interests and expectations. Likewise, if papers preceding yours seem likely to deal with something replicated in your paper, you may choose not to emphasise that area in your discussion. Before you finalise your paper, find out if the conference has a webpage listing the program of papers, so that you can see what other papers will precede yours or be in the same session. You may be able to read the abstracts of other papers in your session, prior to the conference.

(d) The venue and audio-visual arrangements

Conference facilities and audio-visual support vary. Conference organisers will either ask you to inform them of your needs or tell you the range of audio-visual equipment available in the room where you will be presenting. They may even insist on a particular format for presentation (e.g. PowerPoint, on a CD-ROM). Sometimes organisers will send you a plan and information about the seating capacity of your allocated venue. This can help you to decide which audio-visual support you will use.

Developing an effective presentation

You have an attention-grabbing title and an idea of the audience's characteristics. Now you must maintain their interest. Draw on the conference theme and introduce your paper with a short narrative, arresting statistics, thought-provoking quotes, interesting visuals, or a cartoon. Don't attempt to tell a joke unless you have a real gift for humour regularly affirmed by others. However, *do* think about all the boring and irritating talks you have attended and avoid duplicating poor practices (Smith 2000; Gruhn 2001).

Prepare for the ear and the eye

Different health and social science disciplines have different presentation styles at conferences. Medical and dental professionals and medical scientists rarely read a paper. Usually they talk from the points on slides or PowerPoint presentations. By contrast, a policy analyst presenting a discursive analysis of the history of aged care reform may well prefer to present a prepared paper. Whatever the tradition of your field, as a novice you would be wise to prepare speaking notes and practise aloud, preferably in front of an audience of friends or colleagues. It is important to note, however, that oral presentations are not essays read aloud (Bly 2003). They are presentations that are specially structured to present information in a way that anticipates and answers the questions in the minds of the audience. To do this you need to ask yourself what your audience will want to know at various points during the talk in order to maintain their interest and aid their understanding. Use short sentences and omit complex jargon; don't assume that your audience is familiar with your technical language. Give brief explanations of terms that are to be used throughout the talk (Lunemann 2001). Use visual aids to illustrate your points but do not overload them with text. Limit the number of slides and leave them up for long enough to be read. Use your speaker's notes for the information to fill out the key points made on visuals.

Some basic guidelines for structuring a presentation are shown in Table 21.1. Remember that you will need to tailor your talk to the time available. Note that while the guidelines in Table 21.1 seem to advocate repetition, you are not repeating the same words but rather highlighting the key message differently to introduce, detail, and conclude your topic.

Table 21.1 Structuring a presentation

Task	Description
1. Tell them what you are going to tell them.	• Introduce the topic. • State the aims or purpose. • Define the scope and limitations. • Provide an outline of the presentation and the availability of handouts.
2. Tell them.	• Present the key content of your paper in three or four main points. • Use evidence from a variety of appropriate sources to defend each point. • Illustrate each point with examples. • Reiterate and restate the points and the links between them.
3. Tell them what you told them.	• Summarise your presentation as a take-home message. • Provide direction for the audience on how to follow up or use your work.

Introduction

Be clear about the goals of your talk at the outset. Let your audience know about the structure of your talk. Consider doing this with an opening visual that you discuss briefly. You should also define the scope of the presentation. For example, if you were using Figure 21.1

Figure 21.1 Example of an outline visual

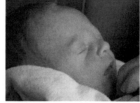

Australian home births: Outline

- Background literature and statistics on home births in Australia
- Research problem: An examination of the health outcomes of home births
- Description of the research study: sample, methods and analysis
- The key health outcomes
  + maternal
  + baby
- Future direction

as your opening visual, you could alert the audience to the fact that, although data are available on maternal satisfaction with Australian home births, because of the time constraints only data on health outcomes will be presented.

Explain the choices you have made about the content you will cover and direct the audience to other sources of information about your work. If you have handouts available, alert the audience to that at the outset of your talk, so they can listen without needing to take notes.

Body of the talk

The body of the session should construct a convincing argument supported by examples from your research or practice. Possibilities for practice-based papers vary across disciplines, from accounts of policy development, educational programs and resources, and practice guidelines or protocols, to demonstrations of practice interventions and uses of specialist equipment. At intervals remind your audience what they have heard and tell them what is coming next. For example, 'I have just listed the physiological challenges identified by people in cardiac rehabilitation programs. Now I want to detail the use of different physical therapies by this group'. Presenters of poorly thought-out talks sometimes find themselves responding to interrupting questions about things they are planning to cover later or not at all.

The Conclusion

The conclusion is the take-home message. It should not introduce anything new but should reiterate what has been covered and offer the audience a way to move forward with the information by reading more about it, following up on your research, or taking action. The goal is to send your audience away with a clear message on, for example, effective strategies for stopping the practice of chemical and physical restraint in the elderly. Don't forget that yours is only one of many presentations that audience members will listen to in the day. You want it to be memorable for the right reasons.

AV Support

Choosing the right form of visual support is essential. In Table 21.2 we have adapted a list of different forms of visual support from Bly (2003) for you to consider.

Table 21.2   The use of different visuals

Visual	What this visual shows
Photograph or drawing	What something looks like
Map	Where something is located
Diagram or concept map	How something works or is organised
Graph	How much there is of something
Pie chart	Proportions and percentages
Bar chart	Comparisons among quantities
Table	A related body of data
Numbered list	A sequential list of data

Research has shown that audiences respond better to combined audio and visual stimuli than audio stimuli alone (Ayres & Ayres 2003). Make sure you are confident in your choice of visual support. If you are told that you must use PowerPoint and you are not familiar with it, then learn it and practise using it before the conference. Likewise, it can be difficult to manage slippery overhead transparencies whilst talking, so it is a good idea to ask a friend to change the transparencies for you.

Rehearsing

People are not 'born public speakers'. Public speaking skills can be learned, but they take preparation and practice. The key difficulties that novice speakers face include 'speed talking' as a result of nerves, trouble timing their talk to allow listeners to hear and retain the main points, and problems using the audiovisual equipment. You can take steps to overcome these difficulties, either through practice and feedback from peers or through professional help. For example, if you are concerned that you will become nervous during presentations and have trouble managing timing, you could go to classes with a professional presenter to practise timing skills.

Rehearsing your talk aloud, with your visual aids, is sensible for a number of reasons:
* It enables you to practise pacing and timing.
* It allows you to hear if you sound stilted, boring, or pompous when moving from the written word to oral speech. (You could tape your talk and listen to see if you need to changes the style of presentation or content.)
* It helps you become competent at managing the material and the audiovisual supports within the set time.

When you arrive at the conference

Make it a priority to check the venue in which you will be speaking. Examine the set-up carefully. How crowded is the room? How flexible is the space? How close is it to distracting noises? Check how much lighting you will have available to read your notes when the lights are dimmed. What is the audiovisual set-up? Can you reach the computer mouse or the overhead projector easily? Will you need to dim or increase the lighting?

Sit in a few chairs around the room to get an idea of how you will look to audience members. If possible, attend an earlier presentation in the same room and see how others cope with the space. Where did the session convenor sit? Did the presenters sit on the stage or in the audience prior to the presentation? Is water provided or will you need to take a

HANDY HINT

21.2 Presenting confidently

* Think about your appearance: make it appropriate for the audience.
* Relax; engage with the audience; don't talk to your notes.
* Be enthusiastic about your topic.
* Speak firmly and clearly into the microphone.
* Avoid long and complex sentences.
* Be aware of the nonverbal messages you convey through, for example, distracting movements of your laser pointer (Munter & Russell 2003).
* Pace your presentation: keep an eye on the time you have left.
* Watch for nods of understanding. If some in your audience look puzzled, be prepared to reiterate your point or rephrase it.
* Conclude strongly and clearly.

bottle with you? Is there a clock in view or will you need to put your watch in a visible spot? Is there a microphone and does that mean you need to stay in one place?

Organise a time to conduct any audiovisual checks with a technician before your presentation. Practise speaking into the microphone or do a sound check of your voice if microphones are not available. Check the lectern and any control buttons. If you are showing scientific or clinical images, will you need a pointer to indicate the key elements?

Delivering your talk

Two (related) keys to effective presentation are to be convincing and to sell your message (Parvis 2001). After all your preparation, this is the time to relax as much as possible and deliver the talk as you have been practising it.

Answering questions

Managing question time is an integral part of every session. Normally there will be a chairperson who moderates questions and makes sure that they are taken in order and that no-one dominates the occasion with their own interests or concerns.

21.3 Dealing with question time

HANDY HINT

- Maintain good eye contact with all the members of the audience.
- If you don't understand a question, ask for clarification.
- Repeat a question briefly if it's likely that part of the audience couldn't hear it.
- Provide brief, clear answers; don't start another lecture.
- Answer to the whole audience, not just the questioner.
- If people make a comment and don't ask a question, thank them for their comment.
- Offer to follow up individually if someone has a complex question or an emotional issue they want discussed.
- Don't bluff if you don't know the answer; admit you haven't considered the issue.
- Allow other experts in the audience to offer ideas or opinions.

Conclusion

Giving a talk at a conference can be a challenging experience, but with good material and careful preparation it can also be tremendously rewarding, both personally and professionally. If you take the time to practise, if you watch other speakers to learn what to do and what not to do, and if you regard your audience with respect but not apprehension, you will be well on the way to giving a first-class conference presentation.

References

Ayres, J. & Ayres, T. A. 2003, 'Using images to enhance the impact of visualization', *Communication Reports*, vol. 16, no. 1, pp. 47–55.

Bly, R. W. 2003, 'Give memorable presentations', *Chemical Engineering Progress*, vol. 99, no. 1, pp. 84–7.

Gruhn, P. 2001, 'Terrified of public speaking? Not anymore ...', *In Tech*, vol. 48, no. 5, p. 84.

Lunemann, R. 2001, 'Oral presentations for technical communication', *Technical Communication*, vol. 48, no. 3, pp. 328–9.

Munter, M. & Russell, L. 2003, *Guide to Presentations*, Prentice Hall, Upper Saddle River, New Jersey.

Parvis, L. F. 2001, 'The importance of communication and public speaking', *Environmental Health*, May, vol. 63, no. 9, p. 44.

Schmoll, B. J. 2002, 'Writing, speaking, and communication skills for health professionals', *Physical Therapy*, vol. 82, no. 5, pp. 524–5.

Smith, R. 2000, 'How not to give a presentation', *British Medical Journal*, vol. 321, pp. 1570–1.

Tyler, S., Kossen, C. & Ryan, C. 1999, *Communication: A Foundation Course*, Prentice Hall, Sydney.

PART 4

INTERPERSONAL COMMUNICATION

22	Leading Groups and Meetings	205
23	Talking with Colleagues, Patients, Clients, and Carers	218
24	Working with Groups: Consulting, Advocating, Mediating, and Negotiating	230
25	Intercultural Communication	239
26	Giving Feedback	247
27	Learning to Communicate Clinical Reasoning	254
28	Working as a Member of a Community Health Team	260

22

LEADING GROUPS AND MEETINGS

Joy Higgs and Mary Jane Mahony

KEY TOPICS

→ Working in groups

→ Balancing group process and task completion

→ Understanding the roles of group members

→ Being a group leader

→ Identifying tasks and facilitating their completion

→ Leading meetings and committees

Introduction

Group work is a key aspect of many of the activities undertaken by students and practitioners in the health and social sciences. In this chapter we address these questions: What constitutes a group? What are the roles that groups and group members play to help groups work effectively? How do group members work together to perform tasks well when they are working in committees and at meetings?

Understanding groups

A group 'consists of a small collection of people who interact with each other, usually face to face, over time in order to reach goals' (Adler & Rodman 2003, p. 256). Baker et al. (2002, p. 320) provide this definition: 'a group consists of people who interact, have a collective perception of their membership of the group and whose activities are structured and interdependent'. Groups can be created to generate ideas (brainstorming groups), solve problems, make decisions, manage areas of responsibility (e.g. committees), perform work roles (e.g. rehabilitation and community health teams), promote personal development, and perform learning assignments (learning groups). Small groups usually consist of three to twelve people. The ideal upper limit depends on a group's capacity to perform its task effectively and for group members to know each other well enough to work well together.

Groups have two major roles: the first is build relationships (to maintain the group and support the group members) and the second is to complete tasks. A number of chapters in this book deal with different aspects of working in groups to enhance interpersonal communication and working relationships (see Chapters 23, 24, and 28). The task aspects of group work are discussed below.

HANDY HINT ☞ 22.1   Group cohesion

Remember that group members are interdependent. Effective groups are cooperative and supportive in good times and when problems arise. As Ellis et al. (2003) have written, 'Effective groups demonstrate group cohesion: they have good organisation, good relationships and good achievement records.'

When individuals start forming a group, they need to get to know each other, to clarify what the goals and tasks of the group are, to negotiate the roles of the various group members, and to set parameters for the group (e.g. time-line and type of product required or desired). In the early stages of group work, the group also establishes norms, or rules, which may be explicitly stated or written down, or implicit and tacitly accepted. These rules and expectations can be divided into *social* norms (governing relationships), *procedural* norms (identifying how the group will operate), and *task* norms (or rules for getting the job done) (Adler & Rodman 2003). Table 22.1 provides examples of group norms.

Not long after group formation, a phase of group conflict can occur, while the group seeks to establish its leadership and direction. After these initial developmental phases, groups commonly focus on the performance of their task roles. Group maintenance and support are still important at this stage, particularly if conflicts or difficulties arise (see Chapter 24). Supporting people is also an important part of finishing tasks, celebrating successes, and winding down the group. A well-known model of group development (Tuckman 1965; Tuckman & Jensen 1977) describes the stages of group development as forming, storming, norming, performing, and mourning.

Balancing group process and task completion

One of the important aspects of group work is finding an appropriate balance between group process and task completion. There can be times when it is most desirable for the group to concentrate on social relationships: for instance, when the group is forming or celebrating, or when some disharmony or confrontation needs to be dealt with. In such cases,

Table 22.1   Examples of group norms

Subject	Examples of issues addressed
Appearance	How formally/informally should people dress?
Behaviour	What sort of behaviour is acceptable? How will the group deal with unacceptable behaviour (e.g. sexist or racist language)?
Workload	How hard should people work? How should work be shared around? What will the group do if people don't share the work fairly?
Social arrangements	Will the group socialise as well as work together? What is acceptable or unacceptable behaviour (e.g. forming cliques, excluding people from social events)?
Allocation of resources	How are tasks resourced? How are tasks and resources allocated?
Punctuality	How important is it to arrive on time? What does the group expect?
Time-line	How strict are the deadlines? Is it essential for all tasks to be completed on time?
Quality of work	What level of quality, quantity, accuracy, consulting, and editing is expected in work done for the group?
Problems in the group	What strategies will the group use to deal with group problems (such as breaking of the ground rules, interpersonal conflict, and stresses or issues that arise in the group)?
Consequences	How will the group reward/punish people if they follow/break the rules of the group? How will the group remind members of the rules?

Source: Informed by Baker et al. 2002

the task roles of the group are being compromised. It can be beneficial at these times to concentrate on group maintenance or social issues, rather than persisting ineffectually or inefficiently with a task, or even making errors of judgement and failing to meet task goals. On other occasions, particularly if a group is working well, it is desirable and most effective to concentrate on task performance and completion, with little (but sufficient) attention to group support. There are times when external parameters, such as deadlines and competing work demands, prompt the group to concentrate on the task. Silberman and Clark (1999) describe a range of strategies to address both process and task needs.

Cultural differences need to be considered, both when attending to group relationships and when focusing on task completion. Factors to consider include individual members' facility with the language being used by the group, culturally influenced views of individuals' and the group's roles and responsibilities, expectations members have of the group leader, the importance of interpersonal relations compared to completion of the task, and whether saving face is important in group situations. There is no single answer to these issues, because cultures vary; however, DeVito (2003) reported research suggesting that one guide is the distinction between individual (low context) cultures and collective (high context) cultures. People from low context cultures tend to act individually, expect everything to be explicit, and do not set high importance on personal relationships. People from collective cultures tend to see the group's goals, values, and welfare as most important, perceive individual roles from this perspective, and value personal relationships and mutual respect. In groups composed of individuals with different cultural backgrounds, the group leader has a responsibility to be sensitive to potential differences in understanding and expectations.

Roles of group members

Group members can take on a variety of task and relationship (or group-maintenance) roles to help the group work effectively. In addition, they may take on dysfunctional roles that prevent groups from forming or performing well. Roles may be consciously chosen, may emerge during the life of the group, may be customary (e.g. based on personality, with some individuals tending to adopt leadership or disruptive roles), or may be assigned by authority figures like teachers or by the group (e.g. by voting). Table 22.2 provides an overview of such roles.

Table 22.2 Roles of group members

Task roles	Typical behaviours
Initiator/Contributor	Contributes ideas and suggestions. Proposes solutions and decisions. Proposes new ideas or states old ideas in new ways.
Information seeker	Seeks clarification of comments (e.g. accuracy of terms or data). Asks for information, facts, and data related to the task or problem. Suggests that information is needed before decision is made or finalised.
Information giver	Offers facts or generalisations related to group's task.
Opinion seeker	Seeks clarification of opinions of others in the group. Asks group members how they feel about (for example) the direction of the group/task.
Opinion giver	Gives own opinion about some aspect of the group (e.g. suggestions made, proposals). Suggests attitude the group should take.
Elaborator/Clarifier	Elaborates on ideas etc. proposed by group members. Offers clarification of or rationales for proposals made. Suggests what would be the outcome of taking up some proposal.
Coordinator	Clarifies relationships among opinions, ideas, information, etc., being discussed. Suggests how ideas could be integrated.
Diagnostician	Identifies problems relating to the group work or proposal.
Orienter/Summariser	Summarises events and outcomes. Seeks to keep the group on track in relation to agreed goals. Raises questions about where the group is heading.
Energiser	Prompts the group to take action or to get back to work.
Procedure developer	Handles routine tasks, such as organising seating, preparing equipment, and handing out papers.
Secretary	Takes notes on group's activities and progress.

Table 22.2   Roles of group members   (continued)

Task roles	Typical behaviours
Evaluator/Critic	Constructively analyses group's achievements according to some standards. Checks if agreement has been reached.

Social roles	Typical behaviours
Supporter/Encourager	Praises, agrees with, and accepts others' contributions. Offers warmth, recognition, and solidarity.
Harmoniser	Reconciles disagreements, mediates differences, and provides opportunities for members to explore differences to reduce tension and promote harmony.
Tension reliever	Reduces tension and formality with jokes or other means.
Conciliator/Compromiser	Tries to resolve conflict between own ideas and those of others; offers compromises. Admits own errors to promote group cohesion.
Gatekeeper/Expediter	Encourages and facilitates input from silent members. Keeps communication channels open by reinforcing efforts of others.
Feeling expresser	Makes the feelings, moods, and relationships in the group explicit. Shares own feelings with the group.
Follower	Passively goes along with the group, accepts ideas of others, and acts as audience.

Dysfunctional roles	Typical behaviours
Blocker	Interferes with group's progress by rejecting ideas or adopting negative stance on issues. Refuses to cooperate.
Aggressor	Criticises, dominates, and puts down other people.
Deserter	Withdraws; engages in irrelevant side conversations.
Dominator	Dominates discussion; monopolises group's time.
Recognition seeker	Seeks attention and recognition at expense of group performance.
Confessor	Expresses own feelings and perspectives rather than focusing on the group.
Help seeker	Expresses insecurity or confusion and self-deprecation, seeking sympathy from others.
Special-interest pleader	Disregards the goals of the group and pleads the case of some special group.
Joker	Displays inappropriate humour.
Cynic	Discounts group's chance of success.

Sources: Based on Adler & Rodman 2003; DeVito 2003

Table 22.3 Leadership style and control

Style	Level of member control and responsibility	Level of leader control and responsibility	Leadership features	Outcomes/Relevance
Authoritarian leadership	Low	High	• Determines group policies • Makes decisions without consultation or agreement • Encourages communication through leader only • Impersonal • Assumes responsibility for group's progress and outcomes • Commands compliance	• Group is not satisfied but is efficient • Can be useful in crisis situations
Parental leadership	Low	High	• Similar to authoritarian leader (i.e. high control), but will listen to feedback • Tends to 'sell' strategy to subordinates rather than 'tell' them • Uses parental types of reward and punishment	• Resented by competent groups and group members • Can be useful for mentoring and supervising novices
Democratic or participative leadership	Moderate	Moderate	• Provides direction but allows group to influence direction • Encourages members to set goals • Reinforces members • Contributes suggestions • Allows group to make decisions	• Group is satisfied and efficient • Achieves group and member empowerment • Can be time-consuming
Laissez-faire leadership	High	Low	• Shows no initiative in directing actions • Relinquishes authority and is often irresponsible • Offers little reinforcement of group members • Provides information only on request • Does not manage problem members	• Group is satisfied but inefficient • Can work when group is self-directed and well motivated

Source: Based on DeVito 2003; Tyler et al. 2002

Being a group leader

Group leaders can be formally elected, appointed by an external authority (e.g. a teacher or employer), determined according to pre-existing professional responsibilities (e.g. the head of a hospital department could be responsible for chairing an occupational health and safety committee), or emerge informally in a group (e.g. certain people could volunteer to lead, 'take over', or gain support of the group members). Leaders should recognise that the value of working with a group is that it can harness all members' ideas, talents, past experience, and work capacity, and so it is not desirable for the leader to dominate a group. Rather, the leader should serve as the overall group process facilitator, promoting effective task, social, and maintenance activities by involving others in these roles.

Leading does not mean doing all the work. It does mean ensuring that goals are reached. If you are a group leader, you need to ensure that:

- the group's goals are defined (including an overall aim and specific objectives)
- the tasks to achieve the goals are identified, explicitly described, and understood by all
- an action plan for completing the tasks is prepared, including specification of tasks, responsibilities of each group member, intermediate and final deadlines, what resources may be needed, how progress will be monitored, and how completion of tasks will be indicated
- a good working relationship is established in the group (i.e. understanding, trust, and effective communication are developed and maintained among the group's members).

To achieve these outcomes, it is useful for a leader to:

- promote a climate conducive to effective and supportive group work
- organise an appropriate group venue with appropriate resources (e.g. seating, whiteboards, and computing equipment) and support personnel if required (e.g. a minutes secretary for formal committees)
- set and distribute agendas and relevant pre-reading materials or minutes
- keep the group on task
- ensure that a record is kept of decisions and completed tasks
- address relationship issues
- be accountable (in terms of reporting and task completion) to the group and to any relevant stakeholders who have an interest in or authority over the group, such as teachers, fellow students, or the community.

Leaders help groups to have direction and be successful. Effective leaders are good role models, work well with people, recognise and value the contributions of others, look at the big picture of the group task and goals as well as the procedures and processes that help to get the task done, share the credit and power in the group, and keep the group predominantly on task. Leaders can adopt different styles, such as being task-oriented or people-oriented. As Ellis et al. (2003) have written, 'Pursuing a single style of leadership may not always be productive in leading a group'. Indeed, it is often desirable for leaders to adopt a series of approaches, at times adapting their approach to their group's needs (in relation to its stage of development and current performance success or difficulties) and at times proactively influencing the group's performance. Table 22.3 describes some different styles of leadership.

Linked to leadership style is the style of communication that is encouraged or emerges in a group. See Figure 22.1 for communication patterns; note the depiction of one-directional versus multi-directional communication (see arrows), relative access to and dominance by the leader, and level of participation in the two models.

Figure 22.1   Patterns of communication in groups

Centralised, hierarchical and closed   Decentralised, participatory and open

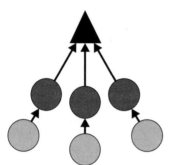 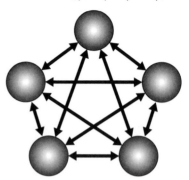

Identifying the group's task(s) and facilitating task completion

Most groups form or are formed to achieve a goal by completing a task or series of tasks. Examples range from students undertaking a group assignment to a project team planning and implementing the construction of a new community health centre. Committees are also groups. They usually have ongoing responsibilities that are broken down into a range of tasks. Examples include management committees of university student associations and the occupational health and safety committees of hospitals.

The group's goal

Consider the group's goal. Does the group want to provide more opportunities for students to have fun on campus? Or is it responsible for vetting all applications for human ethics approval for research activities in a medical centre? The first step is to define the purpose of the group. If the goal of the group is to complete a student assignment, reading and dis-cussing the instructions for the assignment should be the initial steps.

Task identification

What needs to be done to achieve the goal? How you work this out depends on the diffi-culty and complexity of the task. For large tasks, subsets of tasks and stages of achievement (e.g. intermediate goals and time-lines) usually need to be identified. You may wish to start with a brainstorming session. In this session, every member of the group suggests possibili-ties, with no judgements made during the brainstorming. The list is then scrutinised and the merits of items are discussed, similar ideas are combined, and so on. This process works well for high-level task identification (such as the kind of activity to hold to generate more fun on campus). Silberman and Clark (1999) suggest many strategies for helping a group to achieve its tasks.

Constructing a plan

For straightforward projects, a simple action plan may be sufficient (see Figure 22.2). For more complex tasks, the relationships between tasks and the time needed for each task should be spelled out. Baker et al. (2002, pp. 388–93) provide illustrations of several methods for

Figure 22.2 Simple action plan or meeting notes

Action	Who	When	Resources needed	Achievement indicator

visualising the relationships among project tasks and timelines (e.g. Gantt charts and critical path analysis). For example, in a student group project, the plan might include one student, Ying, creating a set of charts using the data provided by the task groups. Ying can't do this until all the data are collected; furthermore, if the data are delivered too late, Ying may not have time to complete the charts. Documenting this in a flowchart (a critical path analysis) will help everyone see what is required. (For very large projects, teams sometimes use special project–management software, such as MS Project, to document, monitor, and report on projects.) The plan also identifies milestones, which can be used by the group leader (or the group as a whole) to monitor progress.

Understanding, trust, and communication

Groups work well when members have a shared understanding of their shared task, trust one another to meet their responsibilities, and communicate regularly about progress, difficulties, and unexpected outcomes. One way of developing understanding, trust, and communication within a group is to hold meetings from time to time that aim to foster communication and build group cohesion as well as complete agenda tasks. Another is to use a range of strategies to support communication and understanding. Keep in mind that individuals vary in the ways they develop understanding and skills. Some people need visual stimuli (e.g. pictures, graphs, charts, and images), some are more comfortable with words and details, analyses, comparisons, steps, and processes, and others may benefit from being able to touch or manipulate things like models.

Problem solving

A common task for a group is to solve a 'problem'. Groups can utilise all the energies and abilities of the various group members to solve problems. Figure 22.3 sets out a commonly used sequence of steps for this process. (*Step 1 caution*: Take time to define the problem, looking at it from many perspectives. Just as a physical symptom is not the disease, but rather an outcome of a disease or other health condition, so the immediately identifiable problem may be only the result of a more fundamental problem. *Step 6 hint*: This could be a real test (a pilot project) or a 'thought experiment', such as 'If we do this, what are the likely outcomes?')

One 'lateral thinking' strategy for solving problems while still taking a systematic approach is Edward de Bono's (1999) 'six thinking hats' approach. Each group member puts on a figurative (or real!) hat which carries the responsibility for a certain type of input to the discussion:

- blue hat = processes
- red hat = emotions
- yellow hat = reasons/logic

- green hat = creative/lateral thought
- white hat = facts and figures
- black hat = cautions and concerns.

Not only does this strategy facilitate balanced input, it also provides a way of managing difficult or shy people by specifying what their input should be.

Figure 22.3 Steps in problem solving

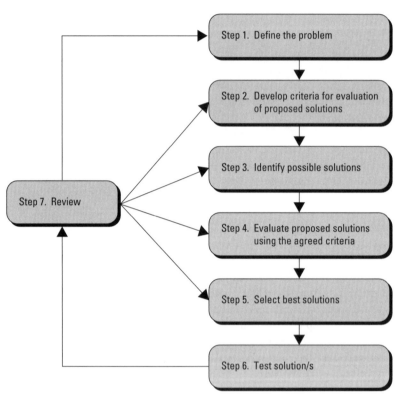

Source: After DeVito 2003

Holding a meeting

Do you need to hold a meeting?

Meetings can be stimulating and productive. They can also be a waste of valuable time, taking time away from professional practice or studies. They are not always seen as value for time spent, particularly if they are poorly managed. Every meeting should have a clear (and explicitly stated) purpose. Of course, there are many possible purposes for a meeting: liaison, group building, reporting, coordinating, networking, task planning, closure, and celebration of achievement (the last kind sometimes look more like parties than meetings). Every meeting requires structure and rules. Some basic guidelines are included here. For more detail refer to Burns (2002), an inexpensive and handy book, or Renton (2000) for a comprehensive guide to meeting procedures, particularly formal meeting rules and processes.

The agenda

A meeting agenda focuses the meeting. From having a list of specific topics, all participants become aware of the scope and sequence of the meeting. The meeting chairperson is also empowered to bring participants' attention back to the topic if the discussion drifts. If prepared in advance and distributed to all participants, the agenda also confirms the time and place of a meeting and any responsibilities for advance preparation and/or leading of the topic. Consider the agenda in Case Study 22.1; what do you think are the strengths and weaknesses of this style of communication?

Emailed agenda for group project

CASE STUDY 22.1

TO: Barb, Viji, Basema, Juliusz, and Ying
FROM: Joe
SUBJECT: Progress meeting on community health centre project
We agreed we'd meet on Friday this week to report our progress and resolve any difficulties. We also agreed to share the load at meetings, so I've suggested names for some of the items. If you don't want to do the task listed, please swap with someone else in the group.

Time: 12 p.m.
Place: Refectory
Agenda:
- Present task reports (Barb and Ying, Viji and Basema, Juliusz and Joe).
- Discuss next stage (Viji).
- Review time-line and plan for putting final report together (Ying).
- Set next meeting date and time (if needed).

Here are some general guidelines on how to prepare a meeting agenda:
- Prepare and distribute it in advance. Having a written agenda helps everyone agree on the purpose of the meeting.
- Consider what item to put first. The meeting may follow an expected sequence, such as dealing with 'business arising' or a series of reports. Or you may put short decision-oriented items first, setting a time limit, followed by a more substantial item that requires considerable discussion. That way you won't run out of time for decision making. Or you could put the most important or most difficult items first, leaving less crucial items to later or even the next meeting. In any event, the chairperson should watch the time used and if necessary negotiate the length of time allocated to specific items.
- Indicate who is responsible for reporting on or leading the discussion on each item. The group should set expectations on the style of reporting (length, content, written and/or verbal report, etc.).
- Indicate any pre-reading expected and how the meeting participants are to access the readings.
- If it is a formal meeting with proposals expressed as motions, whenever possible write the proposed motions on the agenda paper.
- At the beginning of the meeting, review the agenda, adding or revising items and priorities as needed.

Time-keeping

Start on time, keep to the time agreed for the meeting, and finish on time. Everyone's time is precious.

Latecomers

Nothing breaks up the rhythm of a meeting like a latecomer. Usually it is best practice not to stop and bring the newcomer up to date. Keep the meeting moving. If it is a long meeting, however, you could use the arrival as an opportunity for a break, and then update the newcomer privately. If appropriate, also remind the latecomer of the group's agreement about punctuality.

Meeting rules

Your group could agree on using formal rules (see Renton 2000) or informal rules for meetings. Rules may be needed to address:
• how long the meeting will last
• who will speak and for how long
• how decisions will be made
• who will take the meeting notes (and to whom and how they are distributed).

Ending the meeting

You should cover the following at the end of a meeting:
• summary of discussion
• summary of decisions
• summary of any areas still requiring consideration
• review of agreed tasks, who is responsible for each, and deadlines
• setting of next meeting date, time, and venue, if required.
If the meeting is long or complex, the first four points can be carried out at the end of each major agenda item. Finally, it can be useful to evaluate the meeting by asking for feedback. What was useful about the meeting? What could have been done differently?

Meeting notes

As a minimum, the meeting notes, or minutes, should document who was present and what decisions were made. These decisions will include actions (see Figure 22.3). Most ongoing committees use a formal minute structure (formats are suggested in all books on meeting procedures, and are sometimes prescribed by an organisation), while task groups need document only the essential information. If there is no appointed or elected minute secretary, ask for a volunteer. Generally, it is difficult for a single person to be chair of the meeting (managing the processes), facilitator (managing the interactions and group dynamics), and note-taker.

Conclusion

To be effective, a group must attend to both people issues and task issues, and all members of the group must contribute. Both the designated leader and other members of the group can play a part in leading, supporting, and evaluating the group.

References

Adler, R. B. & Rodman, G. 2003, *Understanding Human Communication*, 8th edn, Oxford University Press, New York.

Baker, E., Barrett, M. & Roberts, L. 2002, *Working Communication*, John Wiley and Sons Australia, Milton, Qld.

Burns, R. B. 2002, *Making Meetings Happen: A Simple Guide to Planning, Conducting and Participating in a Successful Meeting*, Allen and Unwin, Crows Nest, NSW.

de Bono, E. 1999, *Six Thinking Hats*, Back Bay Books, Boston.

DeVito, J. A. 2003, *Human Communication: The Basic Course*, 9th edn, Allyn and Bacon, Boston.

Ellis, R. B., Gates, B. & Kenworthy, N. 2003, *Interpersonal Communication in Nursing*, 2nd edn, Churchill Livingstone, Edinburgh.

Renton, N. E. 2000, *Guide for Meetings and Organisations*, LBC Information Services, Pyrmont, NSW.

Silberman, M. & Clark, K. 1999, *101 Ways to Make Meetings Active: Surefire Ideas to Engage Your Group*, Jossey-Bass, San Francisco.

Tuckman, B. W. 1965, 'Developmental sequences in small groups', *Psychological Bulletin*, June, pp. 384–99.

Tuckman, B. W. & Jensen, M. C. 1977, 'Stages of small-group development revisited', *Group and Organisational Studies*, December, pp. 419–27.

Tyler, S., Kossen, C. & Ryan, C. 2002, *Communication: A Foundation Course*, 2nd edn, Prentice Hall Australia, Sydney.

23

TALKING WITH COLLEAGUES, PATIENTS, CLIENTS, AND CARERS

Lindy McAllister and Annette Street

KEY TOPICS

→ Purposes of talking with colleagues, patients, clients, and carers

→ Principles of effective oral communication

→ Strategies for effective oral communication

→ Dealing with difficult communication situations

Introduction

Communicating with colleagues, patients, clients, and their carers is an important professional skill (see, for example, Stein-Parbury 2000, Ellis et al. 2003, Lloyd & Bor 2004). As a key building block for effective professional or therapeutic relationships, oral communication requires care and skill. It must be practised by students and developed further after graduation. Developing good oral communication takes time, practice, and constructive evaluation and feedback from clients, team members, and managers. It also requires reflection and self-evaluation. This chapter introduces some principles and strategies of good oral communication in professional practice settings.

Purposes of talking with colleagues, patients, clients, and carers

We talk with our colleagues, patients, clients, and their carers for a variety of purposes, as shown in Table 23.1. All these purposes are important. For instance, creating and maintaining social relationships is crucial to effective work with clients and colleagues. Being able to correct people and offer feedback is vital for enabling colleagues, patients, clients, and carers to use information

Table 23.1   Purposes of talk between professionals and colleagues, patients, and carers

Purpose	Examples
To inform	• Conveying the results of tests to a patient • Informing a colleague about dates for a meeting • Delivering news of a poor prognosis about a family member to a carer
To educate	• Instructing a carer how to position a patient in a wheelchair • Telling a colleague about a new treatment technique
To correct	• Explaining and showing to a patient the right way to do an exercise • Telling a colleague how to do an administrative task accurately
To negotiate	• Deciding with colleagues who will act as case manager for a patient • Working out with a patient and carer the best discharge plan, given family commitments and medical needs
To support	• Listening to and empathising with a carer about difficulties getting their loved one to eat • Encouraging a colleague who has received a poor performance appraisal
To counsel	• Talking with a carer to help them through their grief over a poor prognosis for a loved one • Discussing with a patient their frustration and anger at no longer being able to drive • Helping an injured client regain a sense of control over the rest of their life
To give feedback	• Telling a colleague how you felt when she criticised your patient care plan at a team meeting • Informing a carer about the progress his family member is making towards their rehabilitation goals
To confront	• Telling a patient that you will not be able to continue treatment if they do not comply with their program • Telling a colleague that you can no longer tolerate certain behaviour in staff meetings
To create and maintain social bonds	• Chatting with colleagues about their weekend • Asking after a patient's spouse or children • Talking to a carer about a family wedding

and achieve their goals. Being able to support and counsel others is as important as informing and educating. Successful professionals in the health and social sciences don't just talk; they also listen effectively (Tyler et al. 1999) and, as discussed in Chapter 26, they provide feedback.

To communicative successfully for all of these purposes, different communication styles are called for. These are discussed later in this chapter. Effective oral communication rests on a number of principles, which we will now examine.

Principles of effective oral communication

Communication is one of the many human interactions that occur in human services contexts. In today's world of quality assurance, evidence-based practice, and accreditation of health and social services institutions, much attention is paid to clarifying expectations of good practice. Communication occurs within this context. In Table 23.2 one example of the setting out of these expectations is presented, in the form of a Patient's Charter of Rights.

Table 23.2 Outline of the ACT's Public Hospital Patients' Charter

Area of Service	Elements addressed in the Charter
Access to services	• Public or private hospital care • Choosing your doctor • Waiting lists • A range of services • Making decisions • Consent to treatment • Participation in research • If you cannot consent • Other decisions
Being informed	• Information about people who are treating you • Information about your treatment • Information about treatment options • Information about services available • Interpreter services • Information in medical records
Being treated with respect and dignity	• Treatment without discrimination • Confidentiality • Privacy
If things go wrong	• Dealing with problems as soon as they arise • Getting the best health care

Source: The ACT's Public Hospital Patients' Charter is a requirement under the Medicare Agreement between the ACT (Australian Capital Territory) and Commonwealth Government of Australia. The full document can be viewed at www.canberrahospital.act.gov.au (accessed 15 January 2004).

A number of principles guide and explain effective communication:
- Communication is not static; it is dynamic and rapidly changing.
- Communication is transactional, not linear.
- Communication is both verbal and nonverbal; we use a lot of body language to convey information.

- Communication involves redundancy (we can work out the message even if we miss parts of it).
- Messages have multiple layers of meaning.
- The message intended is not always the message sent.
- The message sent is not always the message received.
- Communication is culturally based.

These principles are particularly important in communication in the professional context. Oral communication is a complex phenomenon. Any communication act has multiple facets. The grammar and vocabulary we choose to express an idea, together with the pitch, volume, rhythm, and stress patterns we use to deliver it; all affect how our message is received and understood by the listener. And there are layers of meaning or nuance embedded in what we say. A statement as simple as 'I got your report' could mean anything from 'Thank you for your report' or 'About time I got your report—why are you always late?' to 'It's not very comprehensive' or 'I really disagree with your diagnosis and proposed treatment.'

What is spoken is only part of the message (Kacperek 1997). 'Some researchers estimate that 60% of the meaning of an utterance actually comes from our body language' (Minardi & Riley 1997). So, if the simple utterance 'I got your report' is said with the speaker having hands on hips, it may convey irritation that the report was late or a desire to argue about the contents. If it is said with a quizzical look on the speaker's face, it may convey a lack of understanding of what is in the report or disagreement about the contents. How you interpret the utterance depends not only on the sentence construction and delivery but also on who you are, who the speaker is, whether you share a common culture or language, your previous history of interaction, the background and context, and both of your expectations about the communication. Because all these factors can affect communication, the message intended by the speaker may not ultimately be the message received. Effective communication depends on ongoing interaction to clarify meaning and achieve the goal of the communication. In this sense, communication is an active, cyclical, or transactional process (Adler & Rodman 2003). Any utterance may be revisited several times in the course of a communication to make sure it is understood and accepted.

Strategies for effective communication with colleagues, patients, clients, and carers

Introducing yourself, establishing a rapport, using positive interpersonal behaviours, and using active listening are all key elements of effective interpersonal communication (Minardi & Riley 1997). Always introduce yourself and explain your status. If you are a student, make this clear. Check with patients how they want to be addressed; ask if they want to be addressed by their title (e.g. Reverend, Professor, Dr, Mr, Mrs, Miss, or Ms). If they say 'Call me John/Jane', then you can address them by their given name. If you are discussing your clients with other professionals or presenting their cases in class, you should refer to them by their formal title. As a general rule, address older people and people from cultures other than your own by their formal title, unless they suggest otherwise.

Rapport refers to an affinity, a sympathetic relationship or a therapeutic alliance (Sharpley et al. 2000). It is achieved through the use of active listening and positive interpersonal behaviours such as respect, empathy, genuineness, and concreteness. Active listening involves a number of nonverbal and verbal actions that indicate you are listening (such as nodding, smiling, saying 'yes' and 'mmm', etc.). Remember that you need to be sensitive to nonverbal communication if your patient or client cannot speak (even if only temporarily, as during dental treatment).

23.1 Active listening

Active listening involves such behaviours as these: maintaining eye-contact, nodding, mirroring the other person's key vocabulary, modulating pitch and phrasing, gesturing appropriately, adopting an appropriate posture, giving verbal encouragement (e.g. 'mmm', 'uh huh'), paraphrasing, reflecting, summarising, and requesting clarification of what the other person is saying.

These strategies can be practised and improved in a number of ways. Rehearsing or role-playing and receiving constructive feedback in a supportive learning environment is a powerful way to learn or improve communication skills. You could audiotape or videotape (with appropriate consent) interactions with colleagues, patients, carers, or fellow students, and then evaluate your communication style, observing its impact on your communication partner. You could ask a peer to review the tapes, alone or with you, and give you feedback on the effectiveness of your communication. If taping is not practicable you could keep a journal in which you reflect on particularly good or poor interactions. Or you could simply ask your peers and your patients and their carers for feedback on your communication style. This could be anonymous, if individuals feel more comfortable doing it that way, and could occur either informally or as a planned part of an annual performance appraisal.

We work in culturally and linguistically diverse workplaces, and what are considered appropriate communication strategies and behaviours is culturally determined. Something that is considered conducive to good communication or polite interaction in one culture may be considered inappropriate in another culture. For example, direct eye contact and direct questions are used by white, middle-class Australians to demonstrate active listening. But these behaviours may not be culturally appropriate in many Indigenous Australian communities. Less direct means of establishing and maintaining rapport, such as shared activities and seeking information through the sharing of stories, are used in these communities. The power relations between white and Indigenous Australians make the use of direct communication styles even more inappropriate. Intercultural communication issues are considered further in Chapter 25.

Adapting your style of talking

Good communicators can draw on a range of communication styles and behaviours. They do not talk or relate the same way to all people, but adapt their communication to the needs, expectations, and abilities of the other person or audience.

Effective communicators know when to adjust their communication style by judging their communication partner's assumptions and expectations of the interaction, using the rapport-building strategies described above (see also Handy Hint 23.2). Through active listening and empathic understanding they gain insight into the perspective of the other person and get some sense of that person's needs in relation to the interaction at hand. For example, a patient expecting bad news may appreciate it if the doctor initially broaches the topic with indirect, sensitive language. Another example is that of parents or carers who have just been told that their loved one has a terminal illness (Brewin & Sparshott 1996). At that time, they might not be able to cope with an interaction informing and educating them about the medical condition. Active listening and empathic skills are necessary to allow the person to express emotion, and to provide support and counselling. If the relationship between the health professional and patient/carer is ongoing, there will be later opportunities to educate using more technical, direct language.

Good communicators also make judgments about what level of language to use in an interaction. For example, it is appropriate to use professional or technical terminology with a colleague, but not with a patient who knows little of your field. If technical language cannot be avoided with a patient or carer, then it must be explained, and you must give examples of what you mean. It is a good idea to return to the topic later in the conversation, to check the listener's comprehension of what you said and, if necessary, to convey the same message in a different way. The speaker and the receiver thus have further opportunities to check their level of understanding, and can make use of the in-built redundancy in language to develop a better understanding of what is being communicated. You shouldn't just assume that patients and carers can manage only simple levels of communication about their condition; some have a high level of understanding of our fields. After years of managing their own condition, or after researching the subject in books and journals and on the Internet, individuals may have a sophisticated understanding of the relevant professional terminology and theories. Nonetheless, you should always check that people understand what you are saying to them, whether you are speaking to a colleague, a 'naive' individual, or an experienced, well-educated patient or carer.

23.2   Aspects of communication that should be tailored to suit your communication partner

HANDY HINT

- Purpose of the interaction (e.g. to inform or to support)
- Context of what is said (e.g. ask yourself, 'Is this the best time and place to convey this message?')
- Level of technical language (e.g. lay or technical language)
- Directness of language (e.g. when informing someone of bad news, you may need to use an indirect style to 'soften the blow')
- Length of utterance (utterances should usually be kept short, but this is especially important in some cases)
- Complexity of language used (e.g. simple sentences without embedded clauses)
- Mode of delivery (e.g. oral, written, or using an alternative communication strategy, such as interpreted sign language, picture board, or voice synthesiser)

Dealing with challenging communication situations

Adjusting your communication style is particularly important when you are dealing with challenging communication situations. Communication is a complex and often problematic activity. In interactions with colleagues, patients, clients, and carers, many difficulties and challenges can arise. Some of the most challenging situations are as follows:

- communicating with an upset or angry communication partner (as speaker or receiver)
- communicating with a person with a communication impairment
- delivering bad news
- being drawn into communication on subjects outside your area of expertise
- being drawn into collusion with clients
- communicating across cultures
- confronting someone
- delivering or receiving negative feedback.

Communicating with upset or angry people

People who are upset or angry need to have their concerns or grievances listened to before problem solving can begin. Allowing upset people to express their concerns and listening actively can help them to clarify in their own mind the nature of their unease. Knowing they have been respected and heard may allow them then to move on to finding a solution to their problem. Avoid expressing personal judgments; stay focused on the person's problem, not his or her personality. Jointly identify a solution to the problem; an imposed solution is less likely to be acted on and may reactivate the upset or anger.

If you are the one who is upset or angry, you need to consider whether it is appropriate to express your feelings. In some cases it may be, as pent-up negative emotion is counterproductive to an authentic, congruent relationship, and such a relationship is an important aspect of facilitative interpersonal communication. If you express your emotions, do so with reference to the behaviour that has upset you, not to the person's personality or personal characteristics. For example, it is not helpful to say 'You are hopeless—you never do your exercises that I give you.' Assertive communication uses:

- 'I' statements—'I feel angry when …'
- clear references to the behaviour that is problematic for you—'When you don't do your home practice …'
- clear statements about the impact of the behaviour—'… as you will slow your progress and that will affect my ability to discharge you and bring on another patient who also needs my services'
- clear statements about what alternative behaviour you expect—'If you want to improve and you wish to keep receiving services at this clinic, you will need to …'

Assertive communication statements can usefully be combined to make clear your feelings, the actions that are causing difficulties, and the consequences of those actions. Case Study 23.1 gives an example.

23.1 CASE STUDY

Assertive communication with a client

A carer has failed to bring in a patient, Joe, for six weeks in row and has not called you to cancel appointments or offer an explanation. Ineffective communication would be to say, 'I'm sick of your slackness in missing appointments.' Here is an example of assertive and more effective communication: 'When you miss appointments without calling to cancel, I get upset because your appointment time could have gone to someone else who needs it and is motivated to improve. It also means that Joe's progress will be much slower. I understand that sometimes it is difficult to get him to come to the hospital, but if you are to continue receiving our services you must call if you cannot attend an appointment.'

Communicating with people who have trouble communicating

Adapting your communication style is particularly critical when you are dealing with patients or carers who have communication impairments. About one in seven people has a communication impairment (Speech Pathology Australia 2004), so as a professional you will need to be aware of communication impairments and develop some strategies for communicating with people who have problems hearing, speaking, reading, or writing. People are born with or develop communication impairments due to a range of factors, including hearing loss and deafness, intellectual impairment, mental health problems, autism spectrum disorder, cleft palate and other congenital craniofacial anomalies, cerebral palsy, traumatic brain injury, head and neck cancer, stroke, and progressive neurological conditions such as multiple sclerosis and Parkinson's disease.

Many such people can communicate using speech if they receive some basic consideration and assistance from their communication partner. Focus on what the person is communicating, not on how it sounds. Check that they have understood you and you have understood them correctly. Ask if they need assistance, but respect that they may not want any. If they do want assistance, this could be as simple as allowing them longer to get their message across, or providing a pen and paper if their speech is impaired but their writing is not. People with reading difficulties may benefit from having supplementary written material that uses visual cues, such as photographs, line drawings, or symbols. Good examples of symbol-supported text for use with people who have aphasia after a stroke can be found at http://www.ukconnect.org/com-dis/index.html?what. Do not shout at people with communication impairments; they are often not deaf, and shouting demeans you and them. Similarly, do not talk down to people who have communication impairments; they may well have normal intelligence and be able to understand you but not respond.

Individuals with a hearing impairment may require a sign language interpreter or supplementary written material. You will need to ensure that you speak to them in a quiet environment with no background noise or glare, to enhance their chances of hearing and lip-reading what you say. If they have a hearing aid, check that it is on, properly fitted into the ear canal, and functioning. Sit nearer to their side with the best hearing or a hearing aid, facing them so that they can lip-read if they are able. You may need to speak a little louder and more slowly than normal, but do not shout at people with hearing loss; this distorts the speech signal and it is demeaning.

Some people, however, have speech that is unlikely to be understood, or they are unable to speak. These people often use *augmentative and alternative communication* (AAC). There are two types of AAC:

- unaided communication—this includes body language; facial expressions; 'pointing' with one's eyes, fingers, hands or body; gestures; and formal signs
- aided communication—this can be low-tech, using objects mounted on boards, charts, and books containing photos, drawings, symbols, words, or letters (depending on the person's intellectual and physical impairments), which the person looks at, points to, or in some way selects to create a message; or high-tech, such as specialised computers and keyboards, or voice synthesisers.

Most people who communicate using AAC use a combination of low- and high-tech AAC. Using an AAC system tailored to their own needs and physical and intellectual abilities can enable a person with a communication impairment to achieve the goals of communication outlined in Table 23.1. But to succeed in their communication they also need a sensitive, cooperative communication partner. You can support an AAC user by becoming informed about AAC, reading basic websites and texts on the subject (e.g. Bloomberg & Johnson 1991; http://www.communicationmatters.org.uk), and following the advice provided in Handy Hint 23.3.

Communication with people with a disability is a common activity and a core professional competency for health and social science professionals. Some strategies to adopt when communicating with people with a disability are listed in Handy Hint 23.4.

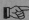

HANDY HINT

23.3 Communicating with someone who uses AAC

- Get on the same level as the AAC user; if they are sitting, sit at their level. It not only empowers the other person, but also allows you to see and use body language to communicate.
- Check with the AAC user how their AAC system works. AAC users usually carry information for new communication partners on how they communicate and how their device works.
- Don't let your anxiety about the unfamiliar situation interfere with your communication.
- Don't anticipate what the AAC user will say, jump in, or finish their turn for them unless they have previously indicated this is okay (e.g. in their 'How I communicate' materials).
- Don't assume that an AAC user will have little to say.
- Remember that, like most people, people using AAC value social communication opportunities.
- Allow plenty of time for the conversation.
- Use open questions to engage in conversation and keep it going (e.g. 'How was your weekend?') rather than closed questions ('Did you have a good weekend?'). Closed questions will probably elicit just a 'yes' or 'no' answer.
- Tell AAC users when you have not understood them, so they can try to rephrase their message.
- Use yes/no questions to clarify their message (e.g. 'Are you asking me where the toilet is?').
- If the person cannot 'converse', give choices to respond to (e.g. 'Do you want water or fruit juice?'; 'Are you asking me about Sue or Peter?').
- Take turns in the conversation, but remember that AAC users may not be able to signal in the normal way that their turn is finished, so watch their facial expressions, eye gaze, and other body language.
- Learn to both read and use eye gaze, facial expressions, and gestures to communicate more effectively.
- Pause often; give the person time to formulate and communicate responses.
- Learn to be comfortable with silence. Western communicators get uncomfortable if a silence or pause extends for more than 3 seconds. For some AAC users, it make take 3 minutes to compose a simple response to what you said.

Delivering bad news

Delivering bad news is a task that faces many health and social science professionals (see e.g. Lloyd & Bor 2004). For instance, a health professional may need to tell a patient that he or she has a life-threatening illness, a poor prognosis, or is not responding well to treatment. At the outset it is important to assess the person's awareness of and reactions to the illness. This will help you decide the best way to communicate the bad news; you don't want to destroy the person's hope. Bad news is sometimes delivered through 'forecasting', or preparing the person for the fact that the results of tests (for example) may not be clear, or 'staging', in which the diagnosis is conveyed in stages, so the person has time to deal with the implications (Maynard 1997). Even when you have to tell someone that they will die soon, you can give them an opportunity to explore their concerns and help them to think through what a 'good death' would be for them. Do not expect a person's emotions and reactions to be

23.4   Communicating with a person with a disability

HANDY HINT

- Speak directly to the person with the disability rather than through any companion or sign language interpreter with them.
- Offer to shake hands when introduced—even if the person has limited hand use or an artificial limb. Using the left hand is acceptable to most people.
- Identify yourself and others accompanying you when meeting someone with a visual impairment. Call the person you are speaking to by their name.
- If you offer assistance, wait until the offer is accepted (or not); then listen or ask for instructions.
- Treat adults as adults. Address a person with a disability by his or her first name only when extending that familiarity to all others present. Don't patronise people in wheelchairs by patting them on their head or shoulder.
- Don't lean against or hang on someone's wheelchair. People who use wheelchairs usually view their wheelchairs as extensions of themselves.
- Place yourself at eye level when speaking with someone in a wheelchair or on crutches.
- Relax.

Source: Adapted from DeVito 2001

stable and unchanging after you have given them bad news. There are a variety of coping styles. Some people appear to readily accept bad news initially, because it confirms their suspicions and their illness now has a name and prognosis. Others may appear to be in denial or act out of defensiveness. However, these reactions may change over time to include anger, bargaining, depression, anxiety, or obsessional behaviour, as the bad news threatens the existing self-concept of the person. Be aware that the relatives also need support and may react very differently from the client.

You may find that you need to deliver more bad news about a failure to respond to treatment when the person is still coming to terms with the overall prognosis, or while the family is disagreeing over treatments. It is always important to identify the most effective supportive resources to help the person face the consequences of the bad news (Lugton 2002). Although you may refer patients/clients to professional colleagues, it is also important to utilise support groups (e.g. The Asthma Foundation), information brochures in appropriate languages, and online information (e.g. http://www.cancer.org.au) to assist people to cope with bad news.

Being drawn into communication on subjects outside your area of expertise

Clients and colleagues might seek your help or advice in areas outside your expertise. Health and social science professionals need to be clear about the boundaries of their expertise and should refer people to another professional if necessary. For example, say you are a physiotherapist and have been treating a patient for many months and educating his wife on how to help him do exercises at home. You have also been giving her encouragement and emotional support as she takes on this new role. Because of the rapport that she has built up with you, she may want to discuss her feelings of entrapment and depression over the demands of looking after a chronically ill husband with whom she can no longer enjoy a normal relationship. Dealing with these issues of grief and loss in any depth will require referral to a psychologist, counsellor, or social worker. You will need to acknowledge what she is saying, empathise, and gently guide her to the point of recognition and acceptance of such a referral. Another common example of blurring of boundaries occurs in interactions between students and their fieldwork educators. Students sometimes share personal problems with their supervisors, who may try to help them using counselling skills. Supervisors can help students to identify the need for professional counselling, but should not provide this counselling themselves. Doing so may jeopardise supervisors' capacity to provide objective, honest feedback and assessment to students.

Being drawn into collusion with clients

Sometimes clients disclose information to a member of a human services team that they ask not be passed on to the rest of the team. There may be occasions when this is appropriate, and informed consent forms signed at the commencement of treatment should indicate who can be told or receive specified types of information about the client. However, there are also occasions when other members of the team do need to be informed, particularly if the information suggests the client is at risk of harm or of harming others. If you find yourself in this situation, tell the client you need to check with your supervisor about the limits of confidentiality between you and him/her. This is particularly important if you are a student. Tell the client that you are a student and are bound to pass any information they disclose on to your supervisor.

Conclusion

In this chapter we have discussed a range of strategies for ensuring effective oral communication in health-care settings. The strategies can be practised and we encourage you to do this, as good communication skills are the hallmark of successful professionals.

References

Adler, R. B. & Rodman, G. 2003, *Understanding Human Commnication*, 8th edn, Oxford University Press, New York.

Bloomberg, K. & Johnson, H. (eds) 1991, *Communication Without Speech: A Guide for Parents and Teachers*, Australian Centre for Educational Research (ACER), Melbourne.

Brewin, T. & Sparshott, M. 1996, *Relating to the Relatives: Breaking Bad News, Communication and Support*, Radcliffe Medical Press, Oxford.

DeVito, J. A. 2001, *Human Communication: The Basic Course*, 9th edn, Longman, New York.

Connect: The Communication Disability Network <http://www.ukconnect.org/com-dis/index.html?what> accessed 8 April 2004.

Ellis, R. B., Gates, B. & Kenworthy, N. 2003, *Interpersonal Communication in Nursing*, 2nd edn, Churchill Livingstone, Edinburgh.

'How to be a good listener' <http://www.communicationmatters.org.uk/Publications/Focus_On/FO_How_to_be_a_Good_Listener/fo_how_to_be_a_good_listener.html> accessed 8 April 2004.

Kacperek, L. 1997, 'Non-verbal communication: The importance of listening', *British Journal of Nursing*, vol. 6, no. 5, pp. 275–9.

Lloyd, M. & Bor, R. 2004, *Communication Skills for Medicine*, 2nd edn, Churchill Livingstone, New York.

Lugton, J. 2002, *Communicating with Dying People and Their Relatives*, Radcliffe Medical Press, Oxford.

Maynard, D. W. 1997, 'How to tell patients bad news: The strategy of "forecasting"', *Cleveland Clinical Journal of Medicine*, vol. 64, no. 4, pp. 181–2.

Minardi, H. A. & Riley, M. J. 1997, *Communication in Health Care: A Skills-based Approach*, Butterworth-Heinemann, Oxford.

Sharpley, C. F., Fairnie, E., Tabary-Collins, E., Bates, R. & Lee, P. 2000, 'The use of counsellor verbal response modes and client-perceived rapport', *Counselling Psychology Quarterly*, vol. 13, no. 1, pp. 99–116.

Speech Pathology Australia 2004 <http://www.speechpathologyaustralia.org.au/library/31_ FactSheet.pdf> accessed 8 April 2004.

Stein-Parbury, J. 2000, *Patient and Person: Developing Interpersonal Skills in Nursing*, Harcourt Australia, Marrickville, NSW.

Tyler, S., Kossen, C. & Ryan, C. 1999, *Communication: A Foundation Course*, Prentice Hall, Sydney.

'What is AAC?' <http://www.communicationmatters.org.uk/Publications/Focus_On/FO_What_ is_AAC/fo_what_is_aac.html> accessed 8 April 2004.

24

WORKING WITH GROUPS: CONSULTING, ADVOCATING, MEDIATING, AND NEGOTIATING

Ann Sefton and Lyndall Trevena

KEY TOPICS

→ Basic strategies for working with groups

→ Asking for and delivering consultative advice

→ Advocacy on behalf of patients and clients

→ Mediation between individuals/groups in conflict

→ Negotiating to achieve an optimal outcome

Introduction

While many encounters with patients/clients are one-on-one, few practitioners in the health professions or the social sciences work entirely on their own. Particularly in institutional settings, it is common to practise as a member of a small or large group or team, possibly as the leader. Your working group may consist largely of health or social science practitioners from the same discipline, but it more likely includes participants with a wide range of different but complementary skills and knowledge. The role of each member needs to be agreed on and made explicit. Specific individual and group responsibilities (e.g. tasks and actions to pursue between meetings) must be clearly determined, whereas many general group responsibilities (e.g. following the group's 'rules' of behaviour) will be established both explicitly and implicitly as the group sets up its norms and patterns of working together. The group will set the goals, decide on the contributions of each member, and ensure that lines of communication are kept open. Some of the activities can be done rather informally; others must be formalised and recorded.

At university you are likely to have a range of opportunities to participate in group activities. You may also choose to study with an informal group of friends. In these different learning environments you will gain skill in communicating effectively with peers in your own profession and in taking on different roles and responsibilities. In workplace settings you are likely to meet practitioners and students from other health and social science disciplines and to observe their roles. If you experience multidisciplinary learning, you will gain first-hand knowledge of different professional roles and responsibilities.

Asking for and delivering consultative advice

Competence as a health or social science professional goes hand in hand with an ability to recognise your roles, abilities, and limitations. One of the most rewarding aspects of working and learning within teams is the sharing of expertise. Getting advice from other professionals can occur on several levels. It may occur between peers and work colleagues, between supervisors and junior staff, or between a particular group and an external source of expertise, such as a government agency or welfare group. Regardless of the level on which advice is sought, there are some key issues that should be considered.

When you recognise the need for consultation it is important to take some time to define your problem accurately. This might involve listing the key issues you are seeking advice about, prioritising them, and possibly grouping them into categories (e.g. problem identification, action/intervention strategies, etc.). Making the effort to clarify your needs at the outset will maximise your chances of finding the information you need. Most people have had the frustrating experience of going to the Web, vaguely typing a couple of words into a search engine to investigate a topic area, and getting thousands of irrelevant 'hits' and hence wasting a lot of time. If you take a few moments to think about appropriate keywords, you are much more likely to get useful results. The same principle applies to seeking professional advice or opinions from colleagues.

Having thought about *what* advice you need, you then need to consider *where* you could and should obtain it from. If your problem relates to a knowledge gap, the best source of consultative advice may be the body of evidence found in the health or social science literature. If you lack experience in searching the literature, consult Chapter 6 of this book. Librarians, teachers, or supervisors may also be able to assist you. On the other hand, you may require a professional judgement, a second opinion, or advice from a specialist; for such advice you need to refer to a professional person with the ability to make professional decisions, not the literature.

Larger groups or organisations may need the consultative skills of external agencies to conduct surveys or interviews, or to produce reports. Once again, it is important to provide such organisations with a clear statement of your requirements, or you run the risk of not obtaining the type of advice and information you need. If your problem concerns an interpersonal relationship, you may need advice from a more senior or experienced person or a counsellor, but they will still need you to articulate your problem clearly.

Can you trust the advice you receive? To determine whether advice comes from a trustworthy source, you should consider whether the advice:

- is independent or comes from someone with a vested interest
- has the endorsement of a higher authority (e.g. a government department or specialist)
- is consistent with widely accepted standards
- contains information collected using valid methods.

Whether advice is trustworthy, credible, and sound also depends on the context within which you would apply it. What works well in some settings may not work in others. You will often need a make a judgement as to whether the advice you have received can translate into your own situation. Sharing decisions (while maintaining client confidentiality) about the implementation of advice amongst a workplace team or organisation is often a good strategy for sound decision making. Providing feedback to your consultants about the impact of their advice may also be appropriate.

For those who are approached to give advice in consultation, there are also important issues to consider. Listening carefully to what is required is essential. You should summarise what you understand to be the advice or information that the person or group is seeking. Be honest about your ability to meet these requirements, taking into account your expertise, your resources (including time), and potential conflicts of interest. Offer to involve other experts if this is appropriate. The way you deliver your advice should be appropriate to the context in which it is sought. Informal oral advice may be the most appropriate form of delivery for an interpersonal matter between colleagues, whereas a written report or letter is best for matters of expertise. It is generally wise to document advice you give.

24.1 | CASE STUDY

Defining the problem and duty of care

Jill is a social worker at a charitable organisation in a large city. The agency has become concerned about the safety of one of its intellectually disabled female clients, who appears to be the victim of physical abuse by her boyfriend. She is reluctant to talk about it with staff and the agency is worried because she met her boyfriend whilst attending their service. At a staff meeting everyone agrees that outside advice is needed. How might they define their problem? Is it identifying the legal rights of the client in case advice is needed? Is it identifying appropriate services for client support? Do the agency staff members need further training in this area? Does the agency need clarification about its duty of care to clients? Do they need advice on more than one of these issues?

Advocacy on behalf of patients and clients

Taking on the role of advocate for patients and clients generally means speaking up for them, supporting them, or interceding for them with a higher authority. People with illnesses, disabilities, and social disadvantages are often in a position of diminished power. By contrast, as a professional practitioner you are often in a position of authority and may be able to act on their behalf in a number of ways. Students should consult their clinical educator, fieldwork supervisor, or teacher before taking on an advocacy role; it may be more appropriate for them to take action than a student. Advocacy may require some level of assertiveness to ensure that your message is clear to all parties (Tyler et al. 2002).

Advocacy can be on behalf of individuals or groups. Patients or clients may need advocacy of a political, social, legal, personal, or health nature. Individual professionals or service

Advocacy options

Jill has looked further into the living conditions of several of the organisation's intellectually disabled clients and has found that many of those with mild or borderline disability do not qualify to have a government case worker, despite the fact that a number of them struggle to live independently. What are her options for advocacy in this case? She can advocate as an individual, writing letters to politicians and raising public awareness through the media, or she can look for organisations that might be able to act on behalf of the intellectually disabled. To what extent do the clients want her advocacy? How could they be involved? How would you approach this situation?

24.2 CASE STUDY

organisations/agencies may act as advocates. Figure 24.1 summarises common pathways for advocacy in health care and social services.

Advocacy for groups of clients or patients often occurs at a political level, but may also occur at a legal or socio-economic level (for example, improving the legal rights and living conditions of vulnerable groups through government and/or non-government agencies). It may also involve influencing community attitudes through the media, a potentially powerful avenue for advocacy. Human service professionals often advocate at this broader level to improve the health, wellbeing, and safety of the general community. Examples of this approach include advocating for smoke-free workplaces, seat-belt legislation, and the use of cyclists' helmets. Professionals with particular interests may choose to join organisations that advocate at this level.

Individual advocacy by human service professionals on behalf of clients may be as simple as vouching for their identity on an application, or as complex as supporting their claim for housing assistance, legal support, or welfare benefits. Individual advocacy can bring with it some risks, particularly if the authority does not accept your claim on the client's behalf.

Human services professionals may also find themselves in direct conflict with their employers if patient or client advocacy challenges or questions the quality of service or management of the organisation or institution. For this reason, many hospitals and consumer advocacy groups act independently on behalf of individuals and groups of clients (e.g. breast

Figure 24.1   Common pathways for advocacy in health care and social services

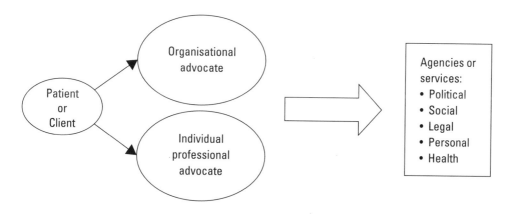

cancer support groups—see http://www.breasthealth.com.au/livingwithcancer/support-groups.html). It is often best to refer patients and clients to such independent advocates, particularly if you see a potential for conflict with your employer. Such advocates will usually be able to provide an experienced and independent voice on behalf of the client.

It is also important to consider the attitude and role of your patients/clients. Do they support your advocacy? To what extent do they want to be involved? Self-advocacy can be empowering, and some would argue that all clients should be involved in advocacy on their own behalf. In some cases this is not feasible or appropriate, particularly for vulnerable groups without resources. It is important to gain clients' permission to act on their behalf, or your altruism may end up doing more harm than good. Your clients' autonomy and self-respect might be seriously damaged if their advocate appears to be taking control of their situation without their consent, albeit with good intentions.

Mediation between individuals and groups

Differences of opinion or more serious conflicts are almost inevitable between members of human services teams, and between patients or clients and/or their families or carers. As a student, you would not normally be called upon to be a mediator in practice situations. However, it is good for you to understand the techniques and issues involved. You may be in a good position to recognise that mediation is needed in a particular case; if this happens you should refer the matter to your supervisor.

The role of mediator is a difficult one and it is not possible to prescribe a set of strategies that will always be successful. But these general principles are a useful guide:

- Use an independent mediator who is perceived not to have a vested interest in the issues or outcomes.
- Provide opportunities for all interested parties to express their views, separately and together.
- Clarify the interested parties' values and beliefs.
- Focus on issues and events rather than on individuals.
- Identify areas of agreement.
- Avoid blaming people if possible and encourage openness.
- Use an empathic approach (try to understand the different viewpoints).

Simple differences that arise, for example in the interpretation of a key clinical observation or in the determination of the most appropriate intervention strategy, can usually be resolved by seeking additional information; you should use the best evidence available. Issues that appear to involve personality clashes, or shades of opinion without a strong basis in evidence, are much harder to resolve. Probably the most difficult are those in which deeply held cultural values or religious beliefs are at stake.

The first step in mediation is to identify the nature and seriousness of the conflicts or disagreements, and to determine where they are arising and who is involved. In Figure 24.2, it is evident that disagreements can occur not only between the patient/client, family, and health-care team, but also within families and within the team. Some even more complex situations for a health-care team also involve outside individuals like teachers or employers.

Once the participants and issues have been identified, it is necessary to gain an understanding of the specific details of the dispute or disagreement. That is often best done by interviewing separately the individuals or groups involved, to gain an understanding of each of their perspectives. It is important to separate actual data from perceptions and interpretations. If the differences have arisen because of simple misconceptions or ignorance, then

Figure 24.2 Complex conflict situations

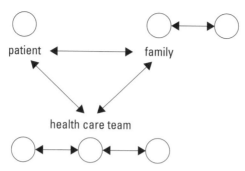

Note: The arrows indicate possible sources of disagreement or conflict.

agreement may be achieved by providing clear, straightforward explanations or relevant data (e.g. in a discussion, by handing out an information sheet, or by directing the parties to an authoritative website or to a patient support group). If significant issues cannot be resolved simply, it is usually necessary to invite the interested parties to participate in mediation or a conference. The mediator is often a senior member of the health-care or social services team, but for serious conflicts an experienced and objective outsider may be needed. The mediator must have a clear understanding of the history of the situation. He or she must think through whether compromise is likely or possible, or whether the situation is bitterly adversarial, making it probable that there will not be a mutually satisfactory solution, but rather perceived 'winner(s)' and 'loser(s)'. If there are potentially serious legal issues involved, the mediator needs to have appropriate training and experience.

Mediation in action

CASE STUDY 24.3

Barbara Bates, who is 84, suffered a stroke that left her with significant disability. She has been moved into a residential unit at the hospital, under the care of a multidisciplinary team for rehabilitation. Her husband, aged 87, is alone at home and is adamant that his wife should be discharged to return home, a view endorsed by some other relatives. The patient herself is unwilling to go home at this stage, although she is worried about her husband's ability to cope. The team believes that not only is she some weeks away from adequate mobility, but home assessment has revealed that some significant alterations need to be made to the home. A mediator in this situation would first establish the facts and perceptions, identifying the key issues by consulting the interested parties separately, and then would attempt to negotiate a compromise acceptable to all parties.

If you are asked to fulfil (or assist in) the role of mediator, be sure you understand the issues clearly. Accurate records of meetings need to be kept. Seek advice on appropriate procedures. One approach when you are acting as a mediator with all parties present is to set the scene briefly in an introduction that outlines your understanding of what has happened. You need to ensure that the parties agree on what are the key issues, concerns, and disagreements. All people involved need to get an opportunity to express their particular perspectives and recollections. The mediator summarises and highlights what appear to be the key concerns, encouraging discussion in the hope that some common ground can be reached. A useful strategy is to engage in a process of question and answer, gaining agreement from both parties on important events, interpretations, and points of principle. It may be possible to negotiate an acceptable compromise, but in some cases it will become clear that one side has a stronger case. Once an agreement has been reached, it must be made specific and endorsed by all parties.

A mediator requires considerable tact and understanding; it is important not to denigrate or belittle any individuals, however misguided their behaviour or viewpoint may seem. Those who emerge as 'losers' must be able to accept that the process itself was fair and reasonable.

Negotiation to achieve optimal outcomes

Negotiation is closely related to mediation, although it need not involve a dispute or conflict. In negotiation there is some give-and-take in agreeing on outcomes and on how best to achieve them. In some situations, a patient or client negotiates with one or more members of a human services team. In other circumstances, effective communication and negotiation are needed between different members of a health team, in order to ensure that there is agreement on specific issues. Negotiation relies on discussion, flexibility, and a willingness to compromise; you must listen to all parties, so as to consider a range of options and ideas. It is a more appropriate strategy than confrontation, bullying, blaming, or passive avoidance of the issues.

Similar skills are needed in negotiation as in mediation. For example, patients or clients (and their families) may be unwilling to undertake appropriate treatments or adopt sensible strategies to ameliorate their situations. To negotiate compliance you will need to be flexible and accept that some goals may not be fully met. There may also be external barriers or inherent limitations that restrict a patient's or client's options. Examples of barriers include financial concerns, distance from experts and/or difficulties in travelling, language barriers, disabilities, fear, and ignorance of the issues. Such obstacles must be made explicit (sensitively) and taken into account, so that the the patient/client and the family/carer can achieve what they want.

In the simplest model of negotiation, an individual patient or client discusses his or her problems with a single professional and negotiates with the professional to achieve an acceptable outcome. When several professionals are involved with a client or patient (see Figure

Figure 24.3 Negotiation involving a patient/client and multiple practitioners

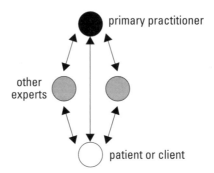

Note: The patient (white circle) consults a primary practitioner (black circle). They negotiate an arrangement whereby the patient is referred to two other consultants (grey circles). Note that two-way communication is focused between the patient and primary practitioner.

24.3), then the primary responsible practitioner usually organises other necessary consultations and advice. Good communication is essential between the primary professional and others who are called in to provide specialist advice. Indeed, it may be necessary for the chief practitioner to negotiate specific issues in the process of referring the patient or client to colleagues.

One-to-one negotiation

CASE STUDY 24.4

Gino Furlan, a 45-year old businessman, goes to his GP for a routine check-up. He is found to be 15 kilograms overweight and his blood pressure is mildly elevated. He comments that he works long hours and has no time to exercise. To save time during the day he eats fast food; he drinks a couple of beers after work and enjoys a bottle of wine with dinner. His GP discusses with him the risks of continuing his present lifestyle. Together they consider how he might reduce those risks. Achievable targets are discussed: he should reduce his weight and alcohol intake to recommended levels. He asks for a referral to a nutritionist and a physiotherapist, who negotiate with him separately an appropriate diet and an acceptable exercise program. Both consultants take into account his attitudes and behaviours, and any physical limitations and other factors that might impair his compliance. They negotiate with him to gain his cooperation in setting and achieving his targets. He will be monitored and encouraged regularly by his GP.

In complex situations (see Figure 24.4), it may be that outcomes seen as ideal by some professionals in the team might not be considered desirable by the other team members. Negotiation will be successful if the team members are prepared to compromise and consider the best overall outcome, rather than the perfect individual (e.g. discipline-specific) outcomes. One strategy is to set out ideal goals or outcomes, and to gain agreement on priorities from each team member in light of the practicalities. It may be necessary to negotiate each goal, setting intermediate targets to provide encouragement to the patient.

Figure 24.4 depicts the situation, common in hospital and community settings, in which a team of professionals works with a patient or client. Negotiation and discussion occur between the team leader and the patient/client, and with all of the members of the team, who each contribute their expertise. Occasionally an expert (e.g. a radiologist) will be consulted without the direct involvement of the patient/client. While the team leader (e.g. the attending physician) carries the responsibility, a great many other members of the team (e.g.

Figure 24.4 Complex negotiation situation

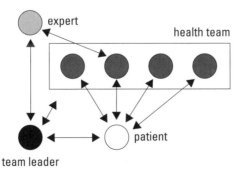

nurses, allied health professionals, medical officers, students) will communicate directly with the patient/client. Those interactions represent powerful resources for the team. However, the patient/client may try to negotiate with individual team members, hoping to gain special information or some perceived advantage. Effective open communication within the team is essential, to ensure that all members adopt a common and consistent approach to the subject. Negotiation is possible only when all parties are prepared to make concessions in order to achieve some reasonable result.

Conclusion

Working with others in workplace groups or informal groups has the potential to draw together the strengths and expertise of a number of people. It can also create problems if differences of opinion or interest arise. The skills of consulting, advocating, mediating, and negotiating are important means of dealing with these problems.

References

Tyler, S., Kossen, C. & Ryan, C. 2002, *Communication: A Foundation Course*, 2nd edn, Prentice Hall Australia, Sydney.

Further reading

Adler, R. B. & Rodman, G. 2003, *Understanding Human Communication*, 8th edn, Oxford University Press, New York.

Ellis, R. B, Gates, B. & Kenworthy, N. 2003, *Interpersonal Communication in Nursing*, 2nd edn, Churchill Livingstone, Edinburgh.

25 | INTERCULTURAL COMMUNICATION

Lindy McAllister and Annette Street

KEY TOPICS

→ The need for intercultural competence

→ Communicating across culturally and linguistically diverse groups

→ Strategies for intercultural communication

→ Working with interpreters

Introduction

Being able to communicate effectively with people from different cultures is an essential skill for human services professionals. It is important to develop intercultural competence, so that you can provide the same quality of care to people from culturally and linguistically diverse backgrounds as to people from your own background. There are a number of strategies that can be learned. You must know how to work with interpreters.

Communication is culturally determined. The way we interact and communicate with people is influenced by our cultural group, as well as by our position within our cultural group. Recall the last client interview you conducted in which you and the client were from the same cultural and language group. How did you introduce yourself? Who was present? What sort of language did you use? Now, consider how you would manage these aspects if you were interviewing someone from a cultural or language group different from your own. Would your interaction differ depending on whether the person was female or male? To manage all these aspects you need intercultural competence.

Intercultural competence

Australia is one of the most multicultural countries in the world. Multiculturalism and bilingualism are features of life in cities and many rural areas in Australia. In the state of Victoria, some 22% of the population either speak a language other than English or have a non-English speaking familial background (Australian Bureau of Statistics 2001a). Twenty-five per cent of the population of the Northern Territory are Indigenous Australians, many of whom are multilingual (Australian Bureau of Statistics 2001b). No matter where in Australia we work as health or social science professionals, we need to be interculturally competent to provide fair and equitable services (see Anderson et al. 2003). The term 'intercultural competence' refers to cultural self-awareness, knowledge of 'the other', and skill in mediating communication (Whiteford & Wilcock 2000). In this chapter we consider how communication differs across culturally and linguistically diverse groups, highlight some strategies for managing intercultural communication, and discuss principles of working with interpreters to facilitate communication with people from cultural and linguistic backgrounds different from one's own.

Communicating across cultures

Aspects of interaction and communication can vary as much within cultures as they do between cultures. For example, the cultural differences between urbanised and traditional Indigenous communities in Australia are marked. In Vietnam, where one of the authors undertakes project work each year, the cultural differences between young, urbanised Vietnamese people and older rural Vietnamese people are striking. Descriptions of the communication practices of different cultures run the risk of stereotyping people, of limiting our understanding of this complex human behaviour, which is constantly in flux, especially under the influence of globalisation, and of ignoring the variability that exists within cultures. Nonetheless, health and social science professionals should still learn about differences in communication modes and behaviour. One series of books that offers valuable insights into cultures is the 'Culture Shock' series by Time Books International (published out of Singapore).

Aspects of communication that vary across cultures are listed in Handy Hint 25.1. The social use of language is one aspect of communication that varies across cultures. Getting the tone of the interaction right is difficult. Striking the right notes of formality, politeness, and directness is a challenge for any of us communicating with someone from another culture. For example, in Western Anglo culture one unspoken rule is that you generally should not interrupt a speaker. Instead you look for the subtle signals that the speaker is about to finish an utterance, and wait for a pause to take your turn in the conversation. Shifts in eye gaze and a change in intonation commonly signal the end of a turn in Anglo-Australian culture. However, this is not the case in all cultures. Further, turn-taking is not universal; in some cultures it is acceptable for listeners to cut into a speaker's turn or talk over them. Variation across cultures also occurs with greeting rituals, such as who introduces whom, how we address someone we meet, who speaks first and last, and whether the verbal greeting is associated with particular gesture (e.g. a bow, a hand shake, or palms pressed together in front of the body).

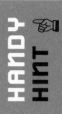

25.1   Aspects of communication that vary across cultures

- Vocabulary
- Grammar
- Length and complexity of utterances
- Level of formality
- Level of politeness
- Level of directness
- Intonation patterns
- Stress patterns
- Pausing (e.g. long or short pauses at the end of a sentence or a speaker's turn)
- Who can speak, to whom, and in what order
- Turn-taking
- Structure of conversations
- Greetings and farewells
- Body language

Interpersonal communication for non–native speakers of a language is made even more difficult by the major role that nonverbal communication plays. Nonverbal communication is the use of stresses, pausing, intonation, and body language (e.g. eye contact and nodding). Table 25.1 shows some aspects of body language that vary across cultures. Nonverbal communication is especially problematic because of subtleties in the way it is used or 'read'.

Table 25.1   Some aspects of body language that vary across cultures

Behaviour	Examples
Touching others	Is it acceptable to shake hands? With men only? Or women too? Is it OK to pat a child on the head?
Eye contact	Should you look at the speaker? All the time? Or should you break your gaze occasionally? Can you look at female as well as male speakers? Is it rude to speak if you are not looking at the receiver (e.g. when sitting in a car)?
Head nodding	Western culture understands vertical up-and-down nodding to mean 'yes' or 'okay' and side-to-side nodding to mean 'no'. The reverse is true in some cultures.
Sitting	It is considered impolite in some Asian cultures to sit with legs crossed rather than with both feet on the floor, especially if the foot of the crossed leg is pointing at someone in the room. Some cultures consider it offensive to sit on a desk or table.
Holding hands	Who can hold hands with whom and in what contexts? Is it offensive for men and women to hold hands in public?
Walking past people	Should you acknowledge people as you walk past them? Verbally or non-verbally? Do you move aside? Which direction? Who gives way to whom on a narrow footpath?
Ways of eating	Is it acceptable to use both hands to eat? If not, which hand should be used for what functions? In communal eating, do you take your share with a spoon or by hand? In small amounts or in one large amount?

Nonverbal communication can easily be misread or misunderstood by the receiver, perhaps leading to offence or embarrassment.

Given the number of cultural groups we come into contact with in contemporary professional practice, it is not possible to have an understanding of the culture and language of every person with whom we need to communicate. But we can increase the chances of successful intercultural communication by being aware that differences exist and by applying a range of strategies to manage intercultural communication (see Williams 1999).

Strategies for intercultural communication

There are many ways of considering intercultural communication. One of the simpler views, used by many professionals in preparation for intercultural encounters, is that of O'Sullivan (1994, p. 99), who suggested that intercultural communication should aim to:
- *avoid* miscommunication caused by cultural factors
- *recognise* when miscommunication could be caused by cultural factors
- *repair* miscommunication that has been caused by cultural factors.

Case Study 25.1 illustrates a failure to avoid, recognise, and repair miscommunication. As you read it, think about how this situation might have been handled differently.

25.1 | CASE STUDY

Problems in miscommunication

Each year a group of Australian health professionals spent a month or so as volunteers in an orphanage for children with physical disabilities in Vietnam. The orphanage had Vietnamese-educated physiotherapists, teachers (not trained in special education), and care staff. One of the goals of the project was to increase the independent mobility and therefore future life options of the children. One strategy for achieving this was to have the Australian health professionals work alongside the local physiotherapists, learning how they managed things and demonstrating different techniques that might expand their repertoire of skills. The chief physiotherapist, Minh, was male and a member of 'the party'. He was often out of the department, but had agreed to the broad goals of the project and was happy for us to work in the physiotherapy department. The other physiotherapists were young females, who were keen to adopt some of the new techniques we share, as they could see their value.

On one occasion, after we had been working with the group for a couple of weeks, we noticed Minh standing to the side watching us and his staff implementing some new techniques. When we asked if he would like to be involved, he said he was happy to watch, as he did not have time just then. He did not appear to indicate through his body language that he was in any way unhappy with what we are doing. We did notice from the body language of the staff that they were nervous, but attributed this to their anxiety to perform the new techniques well. When we returned the following week, the staff told us they had been forbidden to continue using the new techniques

We were perplexed. As the story unfolded over subsequent weeks, we realised that we had been poor intercultural communicators. We had not avoided miscommunication. Although Minh had 'agreed', he had done so to save face. Also, he had not expected that we could show them anything new, and so when staff wanted to take up our ideas, this further added to his sense of loss of face. We also had not acknowledged the power differentials in the culture and the problems that would arise from us showing his juniors, females, the new techniques, and not showing him. We had not explicitly sought his permission to recommend changes. We did not recognise miscommunication when it happened. We did not recognise Minh's lack of involvement and then his facial interest when watching as signs of displeasure. We did finally come to understand the situation and set about repairing it, by ensuring that we maintained Minh's power, status, and authority by getting his assent to future ideas and ensuring his active involvement. Some significant changes in practice and therapy for the children ensued.

O'Sullivan argued that the ingredients of successful intercultural communication are awareness of the significance of culture and its impact on communication, willingness to acknowledge the validity of ways of being, seeing, doing, and communicating that are different from our own, and intercultural communication skills. He identified seven categories of intercultural communication skills, as listed in Table 25.2. Take time to develop these skills, which are useful across the whole range of communication contexts in which health and social science professionals operate, not just with clients from different cultural or language groups. Once you appreciate that communication is a variable human activity, you can begin to analyse and monitor communication interactions for their effectiveness and efficiency, and identify aspects that need improvement. You can also improve your communication skills by being clear, avoiding jargon, paraphrasing, and explaining difficult or confusing words if needed.

Table 25.2   Categories of intercultural communication skills

Category	Definition/examples
Externalisation skills	'Stepping outside yourself and seeing yourself, your behaviour, and your communication from an outsider's perspective' (O'Sullivan 1994, p. 99); thinking about your norms and alternative norms regarding values, assumptions, perceptions, behaviour, and communication.
Analytical skills	Figuring out what has gone wrong (or right) in the communication; analysing differences between the intended message and the delivered message.
Monitoring skills	Thinking about how the overall communication is going: What are we trying to achieve in this interaction? How are the speaker and receiver feeling? Are we succeeding in communicating?
Communication skills	Avoiding miscommunication by preparing for the communication situation; repairing miscommunications; requesting clarification when necessary; avoiding idioms, colloquialisms, and jargon.
Anxiety management skills	Accepting the reality of culture shock; believing in the goodwill of people, aiming to avoid giving offence; communicating effectively and forgiving miscommunications.
Investigative skills	Seeking more information to understand what is happening.

Source: Adapted from O'Sullivan 1994

There are some valuable resources and references available to assist you in developing intercultural competence. For example, Cushner and Brislin (1996) describe a series of critical incidents pertaining to intercultural communication in different contexts. They offer several ways of interpreting the interactions portrayed in each incident and invite readers to reflect on the cultural assumptions and personal beliefs that may underlie each interpretation. As well as reading about intercultural communication, you could seek out a cultural adviser, who can give you an insider's perspective on a culture or ethnic group, and perhaps provide you with opportunities to improve your intercultural competence. Increasingly, this approach is taken in 'cultural orientation' or 'cultural safety' programs for people working with Indigenous communities. Such training is a regular component of induction and training for human services professionals in Australia (Williams 1999) and New Zealand (Spence 2001); it is designed to help professionals provide culturally appropriate services (including appropriate communication) that do not make recipients feel unsafe, uncomfortable, threatened, or not respected. You can learn much by observing how people from the different cultural groups resident in your own country communicate verbally and nonverbally with each other. O'Sullivan (1994) provides an excellent guide to communication between cultures that includes a series of observation checklists to help you sharpen your observation and self-evaluation skills.

Working with interpreters

In your professional practice it is likely that you will occasionally be called on to provide your professional services through interpreters. Interpreting involves translating what is said in one language into another language; for example, interpreting what is said by an English-speaking health professional into Cantonese for a Cantonese-speaking patient, and then interpreting the patient's replies from Cantonese back into English for the health professional. Word-for-word translation is called *literal interpretation* (Isaac 2002). This is often inadequate (and sometimes nonsensical), as it fails to account for the interpretation of words, phrases, and concepts unfamiliar in one or the other language. In addition, culture influences what can be said, asked, and discussed between people (e.g. between males and females) and how disease and illness are construed. Interpretation that is sensitive to cultural differences and aims to preserve the *intent* of the message is referred to as *complete interpretation* (Isaac 2002). As human service professionals we aim to use complete interpretation. Another facet to be considered in interpreting is whether we want simultaneous or consecutive interpretation. With simultaneous interpretation, the interpreter translates while the speaker continues to deliver the message for translation. This is a difficult task for the interpreter, requiring high-level skills, such as those seen in diplomatic missions. More commonly, consecutive interpreting is used: the speaker delivers a sentence or two, pauses for the interpreter to interpret, and then continues with the next part of the message.

Effective interpreting requires a qualified interpreter, one who is accredited (in Australia) with the National Authority for the Accreditation and Training of Interpreters, and who is conversant with the health-care or social services setting and the relevant language (e.g. medical terminology) as well as with the culture of the patient. It is possible for an interpreter to speak the same language as a patient but not be familiar with his or her particular culture (think of the many countries in which Spanish is spoken), so check the cultural background of both the patient and interpreter when booking an interpreter. Sometimes a qualified interpreter is not available. It might be possible to use a telephone interpreter service, or you might have to resort to using an untrained interpreter, perhaps a family member, a member of staff at the health-care facility, or a community member. Be aware that there are major problems with using untrained interpreters, and it contravenes many health institution policies. Family members acting as interpreter may:

- be unfamiliar with the protocols of interpreting (how the professional, patient, and interpreter are to interact; how to clarify communication breakdowns; and so on)
- not understand your professional terminology, nor have the vocabulary for these concepts in the other language
- be unable to interpret at the rate required
- censor, misunderstand, or even deliberately mistranslate what they interpret, or refrain from interpreting all of what you or the patient says
- take over from you or exclude one party from the interaction, perhaps providing a summary of what they believe you want or need to know.

Further, patients may not feel comfortable discussing sensitive or personal information in front of people who they know, or who differ from them in age, gender, or social class. You could end up with incomplete or inaccurate information.

25.2   Working with an interpreter

HANDY HINT

In working with an interpreter, make time for a briefing before the client arrives and for debriefing afterwards. Check that your interpreter understands:
- the purpose of the interview
- the terminology you will use
- what to do if things go awry.

Be clear about whether you want a word-for-word interpretation ('literal interpretation') or a summary that gives the essence and intent of the message ('complete interpretation').

Effective interpreting requires adequate briefing between the practitioner and the interpreter. Isaac (2002) suggested a range of topics for discussion and negotiation with the interpreter before the client arrives. Allowing sufficient time is critical for successful use of interpreters in providing human services. Because of the time taken to interpret, a session with a client that requires interpretation will take longer than a normal interaction. You need to plan for this in scheduling your diary for the day, and you may need to schedule more than one session with a client and interpreter to complete the task (e.g. to complete a thorough assessment or provide adequate counselling). In addition, it is wise to book the interpreter to arrive 15 minutes ahead of the client and to allow time after the client has left to review the session with the interpreter. This post-session debriefing give you a chance to discuss problems in the interaction between the two of you, to identify communication breakdowns or difficulties between you and the client or the interpreter and the client, and to agree on strategies for improving future interactions. It also a good opportunity for the interpreter to act as a cultural informant. The debriefing is especially important if you are likely to work regularly with a particular interpreter or cultural group.

Conclusion

Because of worldwide changes in demographics in recent decades, you need to be culturally competent no matter where you work as a health or social sciences professional. In this chapter we have highlighted aspects of communication that vary between and within cultures, and suggested strategies for effective intercultural communication and for working with interpreters in health-care settings.

References

Anderson, L. M., Scrimshaw, S. C., Fullilove, M. T., Fielding, J. E. & Normand, J. (Task Force on Community Preventive Services 2003), 'Culturally competent healthcare systems: A systematic review', *American Journal of Preventive Medicine*, vol. 24 (3S), pp. 68–79.

Australian Bureau of Statistics 2001a, *2001 Census Basic Community Profile: A Snapshot of Victoria*, Australian Bureau of Statistics, Canberra.

Australian Bureau of Statistics 2001b, *2001 Census Basic Community Profile: A Snapshot of the Northern Territory*, Australian Bureau of Statistics, Canberra.

Cushner, K. & Brislin, R. 1996, 2nd edn, *Intercultural Interactions: A Practical Guide*, Sage, Thousand Oaks, California.

Isaac, K. 2002, *Speech Pathology in Cultural and Linguistic Diversity*, Whurr, London.

O'Sullivan, K. 1994, *Understanding Ways: Communicating Between Cultures*, Hale & Iremonger, Sydney.

Spence, D. G. 2001, 'Prejudice, paradox, and possibility: Nursing people from cultures other than one's own', *Journal of Transcultural Nursing*, vol. 12, no. 2, pp. 100–6.

Whiteford, G. E. & Wilcock, A. A. 2000, 'Cultural relativism: Occupation and independence reconsidered', *The Canadian Journal of Occupational Therapy*, vol. 67, no. 5, pp. 324–36.

Williams, R. 1999, 'Cultural safety: What does it mean for our practice?', *Australian and New Zealand Journal of Public Health*, vol. 23, no. 2, pp. 213–4.

Further reading

Brislin, R. 2000, *Understanding Culture's Influence on Behavior*, 2nd edn, Harcourt College Publishers, Fort Worth, Texas.

DeVito, J. A. 2001, *Human Communication: The Basic Course*, 9th edn, Longman, New York.

Windschuttle, K. & Elliott, E. 1999, *Writing, Researching, Communicating: Communication Skills for the Information Age*, 3rd edn, McGraw Hill, Sydney.

26 | GIVING FEEDBACK

Lindy McAllister

KEY TOPICS

→ Who do we give feedback to?

→ Why do we give feedback?

→ What are the different styles of giving feedback?

→ What are principles of giving effective feedback?

→ What factors/techniques influence the success of feedback?

Introduction

Giving feedback to others is a key life skill. It is an essential skill for building and maintaining pleasant social and professional relationships, for achieving goals for clients, carers, and service delivery and project teams, and for learning at university. It is one of the core professional skills used with colleagues, patients, and carers. While all communication is complex and potentially problematic, giving feedback is even more so. Giving feedback that preserves dignity and facilitates ongoing communication between the communication partners, but

247

that also leads to behavioural change, is a challenge. It requires self-awareness, awareness of others, and of understanding of the principles and strategies for giving feedback.

Health and social science professionals provide feedback to and receive feedback from a wide range of people in health-care contexts, including:

- colleagues
- students
- managers/supervisors
- patients
- carers/families
- stakeholders
- consultants
- funding bodies
- support staff
- themselves

Purposes of feedback

The purposes of feedback vary, depending on who is giving and receiving it. This chapter focuses particularly on giving feedback on a one-to-one basis for the purposes of:

- affirming or encouraging another person
- correcting skills being learned
- confronting someone about their behaviour.

Table 26.1 lists common purposes of feedback and provides some illustrations of these purposes.

Dimensions of feedback

DeVito (2001) described five dimensions of feedback, which can be thought of as continua:

1 positive —— negative
2 immediate —— delayed
3 supportive —— critical
4 person-focused —— message-focused
5 low monitoring —— high monitoring.

This chapter considers the first three of these dimensions. Chapter 23 deals with the importance of a person-focused approach to communication. The 'low monitoring/high monitoring' dimension refers to the difference between feedback that is honest, reactive, and spontaneous, with little self-monitoring or monitoring of the reactions of the other person, and feedback that is deliberate and considered, perhaps provided after a period of reflection and self-censoring, and that is subtly adapted in response to the other person's reactions to it.

Characteristics of effective, constructive feedback

Giving positive feedback is generally easier than giving feedback that is likely to be seen as critical. However, 'negative' feedback can be given in a constructive rather than destructive manner. The characteristics of effective, constructive feedback are listed in Handy Hint 26.1. You can see some of these characteristics illustrated in the examples in Table 26.1.

Even when the main message in your feedback is going to be a correction or recommendation for changing behaviour, begin by saying something positive and specific about what you have observed. People appreciate encouragement. And when you talk about the aspects of behaviour that were not so good, try to include positive suggestions for change.

Assertive and confronting communication

Not all feedback that we give and receive is positive, supportive, or encouraging. While most of the behavioural change we want to foster in our students, in our patients and their families, and in our colleagues and team members can be achieved using positive feedback, there are times when that is not enough. When direct instruction and coaching have been tried and have failed, we have a duty to confront our students, patients, carers, and colleagues if their behaviour is impeding learning, quality care, or professional relationships.

The last example in Table 26.1, that of confrontation, illustrates the principles of providing good feedback even when the message is a 'bad' one. Unlike the majority of the feedback that we give, the feedback in this example is not positive and encouraging. However, it is

Table 26.1   Examples of reasons for giving feedback

Purpose	Example
To provide feedback to someone learning a new skill	An occupational therapist giving feedback to a rehab patient relearning self-care skills after a stroke: 'Mr Jones, you did manage to seat yourself quite well, but next time try sitting closer to the rail. Let me show you. Can you see the difference between what you did and what I did? Can you tell me what the difference was?'
To reinforce skills	A speech pathologist with a child with a speech impairment: 'Great, Peter, you said that really well! I could see that you thought about where you put your tongue that time.'
To provide feedback on behaviour	A team leader giving feedback to a new graduate: 'Susan, it's not appropriate to share personal details about your clients in the tea room. It breaks our code of ethics and infringes legislation regarding privacy. It's okay to seek advice from your colleagues about client management, but you need to do it in a confidential setting and in a way that respects your clients and preserves their anonymity.'
To encourage	A dentist giving feedback to a patient: 'Mrs Wang, I can see that you've been making a real effort to improve the way you brush your teeth and floss. Well done. Your gums are looking much healthier. Keep it up!'
To affirm	A health professional talking to a colleague: 'I like your positive attitude towards this. You are wonderful to work with on this (activity, project, etc.).'
To confront	A manager to a member of staff (or a fieldwork educator to a student) who is repeatedly late in submitting reports, despite receiving previous feedback on this matter: 'When you don't complete your reports on time, I feel angry and anxious: angry because as your manager [or fieldwork educator] I'm the one responsible for problems arising from the absence of treatment guidelines for our patients provided in your reports, and anxious because without your reports the team can't coordinate the management plans and patients can't receive quality care. If you want to continue to work here after your probationary period expires [or pass this fieldwork placement], you need to have your reports in on time or notify me if there is a reasonable delay. I have noted your tardiness in your file and will review your progress towards meeting the report timelines at our next review meeting. If you need help with report writing, please make an appointment to see me or another colleague. I am happy to review draft reports at any time and provide feedback on them. Is there anything further you would like to say about this matter? Would you like me to explain anything further?'

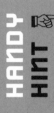

26.1 Characteristics of effective feedback

Effective feedback is:
- sufficient
- specific
- timely
- regular
- encouraging
- relevant
- reciprocal
- not unexpected
- inclusive of recommendations for improvement
- provided when the events/behaviours being discussed are fresh in the giver's and receiver's minds
- related to behaviours that can be changed
- focused on specific problems rather than generalisations
- focused on behaviour not personality
- focused on decisions and actions rather than assumed intentions
- based on first-hand experience and objective data rather than second-hand reports and subjective information

Source: Adapted from Best & Rose 1996, pp. 26–7

still constructive rather than destructive (as it could have been if the manager/supervisor had simply vented his or her emotions and criticised the personal inadequacies of the other person). The manager/supervisor has previously raised the matter of tardy reports, so the feedback is not unexpected and is timely. The feedback is relevant to good health care, and is specific in stating the problem and what needs to be done to improve the situation. It focuses on a behaviour of which the manager/supervisor has personal experience, and which can be changed, and it is not personal or related to personality.

As well as observing principles of good feedback, the manager/supervisor in the example has also used the principles of assertive communication (see also Chapter 23). These principles are to use:
- 'I' statements (e.g. 'I feel angry/anxious …')
- clear references to problematic behaviours (e.g. 'When you don't complete your reports on time …')
- clear statements about the impact of the behaviour (e.g. '… because I worry about the legal consequences of this, for which I am ultimately responsible')
- clear statements of what alternative behaviour is expected (e.g. 'You must have your reports in on time or notify me if there is a reasonable delay').

In addition, the manager/supervisor has:
- offered support to achieve the desired behaviour ('If you need help with report writing, please make an appointment to see me or another colleague. I am happy to review draft reports at any time and provide feedback on them.')
- outlined the consequences ('If you want to continue to work here after your probationary period expires, you will need to …')

- invited feedback and continued communication about the matter ('Is there anything I don't understand or know about what makes this a problem for you? Is there anything further you would like to say about this matter? Do I need to explain anything?')

Factors influencing feedback

Handy Hint 26.2 lists factors that can influence how feedback is given and received. Some of these factors need to be negotiated between giver and receiver, such as the timing, frequency, and location of feedback. Others are background factors for consideration.

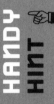

26.2 Factors that can influence how feedback is given and received

- Previous feedback
- Timing of feedback
- Frequency of feedback
- Location of feedback
- Content/nature of feedback
- Goal of feedback
- Readiness and robustness of the person receiving feedback
- Intent and expectations of those giving and receiving the feedback
- Nature of the relationship between those giving and receiving feedback
- Gender and power relations
- Type of feedback

HANDY HINT

Previous feedback

If you have previously given someone feedback about something, then a framework for the interaction and some understanding of the intent and content of the feedback should be in place. If feedback is being given or received in interaction within a new group or pair of people, then rapport building, clarification of intent and purpose, and checking for comprehension of feedback need to take place.

Timing of feedback

One of the characteristics of effective feedback is that it is provided as close to the relevant event as possible. It is difficult for people to recall their behaviour if it took place some time ago. This is particularly the case if people are learning something new or complex, or if they are anxious about their learning or performance. Further, sufficient time needs to be allowed for people to discuss and clarify the content and implications of feedback. In addition, the timing of feedback needs to take into account a person's emotional state. If either the giver or the receiver of feedback is upset, angry, fatigued, or overtly resistant, it would be wise to find another time. Receivers of feedback should feel empowered to say if the timing is not right for them. However, postponement of confrontation needs careful thought, as the timing may never feel right for either party, but it may nonetheless need to be done.

Frequency of feedback

Feedback works best if it is frequent enough to help people make immediate changes to their behaviour. It needs to be frequent enough to build incrementally towards long-term behavioural change and to be supportive for the receiver. Frequent feedback is important for behaviours that affect the welfare or safety of others. For example, if you are teaching a therapy assistant a technique for working with patients, frequent feedback is needed initially as you observe the assistant working with patients. Similarly, if you are running an occupational health promotion program for staff working in aged care, or focusing on safe transfers of patients from bed to wheelchair, you will need to instruct, assist, observe, and provide feedback several times before learners are able to do the tasks safely. Frequency of feedback may need to be negotiated between the giver and receiver.

Location for giving feedback

Feedback should generally be delivered in a quiet, private location, especially if the content is likely to be upsetting, or the giver or receiver is already upset. Feedback given 'on the run' in the corridor, nurses' station, team office, or staff room is not appropriate, unless the feedback is intended to praise or give a public boost to the receiver.

Content/nature of feedback

The delivery of feedback that is complex in nature, likely to require clarification and discussion, or likely to be upsetting needs to be planned. Consideration must be given to how, when, and where to deliver it. Time should be made available soon after the initial discussion for clarification and follow-up discussion. Complex feedback may also require written or visual supplementation, such as a videotape review of behaviours, or written notes supplementing oral feedback.

Goal of feedback

The aim of feedback can be to achieve immediate behavioural change or to work towards change in the future. If the goal is immediate change, consideration must be given to the location and content of the feedback. Who else should be present (e.g. patients or team members)? Does the location offer privacy? Location is especially important if the feedback is not positive or if you are uncertain about the readiness of the person to receive it.

Readiness and robustness of the person receiving feedback

Sometimes people are just not yet ready to receive feedback. They may have a negative mindset towards the giver of the feedback or the likely content; they may be tired, embarrassed, upset, or angry. The giver of the feedback needs to judge the receiver's degree of readiness and make decisions accordingly. For example, if a patient or carer is upset or having trouble accepting the severity and poor prognosis of an illness, it would be better to wait until a time when they feel more receptive to feedback and more able to deal with it emotionally. If a new team member is embarrassed about delivering a poor service to a client, it may be best to leave her time to reflect on the matter and compose herself before debriefing with the manager/supervisor.

Intent and expectations of the persons giving and receiving feedback

When we give feedback, we need to be clear about our motivations for doing so, about whether we have stayed within boundaries that are both professional and appropriate for the other person, and about our own emotions and their impact on what we say and how we say it. Similarly, when we receive feedback we need to be clear about our expectations. Remember, the message received may not be the message actually delivered, let alone the message intended.

Nature of the relationship between persons giving and receiving feedback

Power and gender relations can colour how feedback is delivered and received. Workplace supervisors, clinical educators, lecturers, and professional seniors hold authority by virtue of their position, as well as personal authority. If the giver and receiver of feedback do not share a common first language or culture, power differences can be further exaggerated.

Gender also commonly influences how feedback is given and received. In general terms, when women deliver feedback they are more likely to be aware of the impact of that feedback on the persons involved and their relationships with them, and to try to preserve the relationships by using language that softens the message (Gilligan 1993). When men deliver feedback it may be done in a manner that makes less accommodation for preserving relationships. When power and gender differences combine, the giver of feedback needs to take special care in delivering the feedback.

Familiarity can be both a help and a hindrance in giving feedback. It can be hard to deliver feedback to a friend or someone in a 'dependency' relationship. Old but important work on the games people play in relationships generally (Berne 1966) and in supervisory relationships in particular (Kadushin 1968; Sleight 1984) is still relevant in helping professionals understand difficult interactions with colleagues, clients, and students. Managers and clinical educators should take care to avoid being caught in 'games' (e.g. 'I'm your friend, so you can't criticise me') that make delivering honest, timely feedback difficult.

Type of feedback

Feedback can be delivered orally, in writing, or using a combination of both. Although it takes more time, there are significant advantages to using written feedback. By reviewing it before giving it, you can reach a balance of positive and negative feedback. The receiver is less likely to 'hear only the negatives' and can refer back to written feedback for detail that may have been missed in the emotion of the moment of hearing oral feedback. If feedback is designed to support instruction on a task, then written feedback is particularly helpful. Feedback can also be derived from reviews of videotapes and audiotapes, and from self-evaluations.

Conclusion

In this chapter I have considered many of the factors that can help make the provision of feedback to students, colleagues, clients, and carers a positive experience for all parties. Giving (and indeed receiving) feedback is a skill that needs continued practice and monitoring.

References

Berne, E. 1966, *Principles of Group Treatment*, Oxford University Press, New York.
Best, D. & Rose, M. 1996, *Quality Supervision: Theory and Practice for Clinical Supervisors*, Saunders, London.
DeVito, J. 2001, *Human Communication: The Basic Course*, 9th edn, Longman, New York.
Gilligan, C. 1993, *In a Different Voice: Psychological Theory and Women's Development*, 2nd edn, Harvard University Press, Cambridge, Massachusetts.
Kadushin, A. 1968, 'Games people play in supervision', *Social Work*, vol. 18, pp. 23–32.
Lloyd, M. & Bor, R. 1999, *Communication Skills for Medicine*, Churchill Livingstone, London.
Sleight, C. 1984, 'Games people play in clinical supervision', *Asha*, vol. 26, pp. 27–9.

27 | LEARNING TO COMMUNICATE CLINICAL REASONING

Joy Higgs and Lindy McAllister

KEY TOPICS

→ The nature of clinical reasoning

→ How to communicate reasoning, taking into account audience, needs, and goals

Introduction

Clinical reasoning is central to clinical practice. Health professionals often need to make decisions based on their professional knowledge and judgment in situations where there are no right answers, and where textbook and research knowledge is insufficient or needs to be adapted to the particular patient and circumstances. This is a key aspect of being a professional. The process of reasoning drives practice decisions and actions. Clear communication of reasoning enables patients and clinicians to work together and helps teams to function effectively.

Clinical reasoning includes 'micro' decisions, such as 'What questions do I need to ask this patient?' and 'How does this patient envisage their future after this accident?', and 'macro' (or major) decisions, such as 'What are this patient's major problems?', 'What is this patient's diagnosis and prognosis?', and 'What is the best management plan for this patient?' Clinical reasoning also includes the 'meta' thinking and decision making that you will constantly undertake during practice as you monitor your thinking. For instance, you will ask yourself, 'How do I know if the answer the patient just gave me is complete?', 'Did she understand my question?', 'How well can I do that test, and can I trust my findings?' 'Do I understand enough about this person and this condition to make a sound decision about care?', and 'Do I need help here?'

The nature of clinical reasoning

'Clinical reasoning' is a broad term denoting the thinking, reasoning, and decision making that are involved in clinical practice. At times, for instance when the setting is more community-based than clinical, it is preferable to speak of 'professional decision making' and 'professional practice'. Because clinical reasoning is not a readily observable phenomenon (even though you can see and hear people talking about it and see the results of their decisions), researchers and clinicians have sought to understand it through their research and theoretical models (see Higgs & Jones 2000).

The *hypothetico-deductive reasoning* model (Elstein et al. 1978, 1990) portrays clinical reasoning as a process of establishing hypotheses (e.g. provisional diagnoses and ideas for treatment), testing them by gathering data (e.g. during history taking, physical examination, medical tests, and treatment), and analysing these data. See Figure 27.1 for a diagram of this model. Hypothetico-deductive reasoning occurs in a number of professions, including medicine, physiotherapy, occupational therapy, dentistry, and nursing. It is a thorough, careful process frequently used by novices and by more experienced practitioners working with unusual or difficult cases.

Figure 27.1   Hypothetico-deductive reasoning

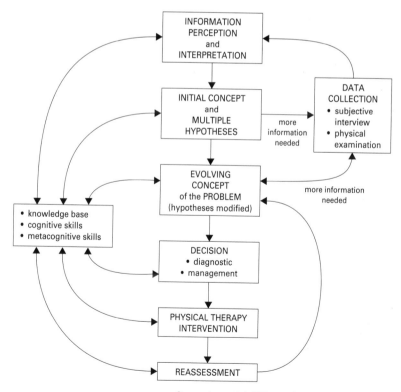

Source: Jones et al. 1995; reproduced with the permission of M. Jones

Pattern recognition (Groen & Patel 1985) is a more rapid process in which experienced clinicians directly retrieve existing knowledge from their rich, discipline-specific knowledge bases in situations where they are familiar with the type of case or condition being considered.

Knowledge–reasoning integration is a model of clinical reasoning that emphasises the interdependence of knowledge and reasoning throughout the reasoning process (see Schmidt et al. 1990).

Newer models of clinical reasoning have been developed, particularly in nursing, occupational therapy, and physiotherapy, to reflect the growing emphasis on patient-centred care and the 'wellness' model (e.g. Fleming 1991; Jones 1992; Fonteyn 1995). Here are descriptions of some of these approaches (Higgs 2003):

- *Interactive reasoning* occurs when dialogue in the form of social exchange is used to enhance or facilitate the assessment–management process. This reasoning provides an effective way of understanding the context of the patient's problem and creating a relationship of interest and trust.
- *Narrative reasoning* involves the use by practitioners of stories of past or present patients to help themselves and their patients to further understand and manage a clinical situation. Practitioners can use such real-life scenarios to enhance the credibility of the advice or explanations they give to patients. Narrative reasoning can also involve the practitioner and/or the patient constructing a future story of the patient's life after an illness or with a disability, as well as reconnecting the patient to his or her life story.
- *Ethical/pragmatic reasoning* is used by practitioners to make decisions regarding moral, political, and economic dilemmas, such as deciding how long to continue a patient's treatment.

Communicating in clinical reasoning

From this discussion of clinical reasoning it is evident that the first person you actually communicate with in clinical reasoning is yourself. This is a good place to start thinking about communication in clinical reasoning, because thinking about one's thinking occurs at a rapid rate, in ideas rather than sentences, often in a rather subconscious way. You do it to assess and regulate your thinking and check for reasoning errors, and so hopefully to avoid making errors in practice (e.g. making the wrong diagnosis, providing inappropriate intervention or care).

By comparison, when you communicate with your colleagues you are seeking to clearly explain something, justify your critique, or get feedback on your reasoning (e.g. what you are thinking about doing for and with this patient). This reasoning, therefore, needs to be clear, in sentence form, supported by credible evidence, and relevant to the task and audience. You will frequently use professional jargon and abbreviations (e.g. BP and CVP) when talking with your colleagues. Remember that such jargon is a tool, a useful shorthand or common language, when you are talking to your peers, but a confusing and distancing barrier when you are talking with patients or other professionals who do not speak the same language. When you are presenting a case at a staff seminar, you would use different language (such as more formal and more detailed explanations) than when you are conversing in a ward with a colleague to share information about a patient.

Your language and communication style will vary again when you are talking with a patient or client or with family members or caregivers. It is often helpful to put yourself in their place. Questions they might be wanting to ask include the following: What do I need to know about my condition or my care? Why do they want me to do this? What aren't they telling me: do I have some terrible condition? Why are they treating me like an idiot?

Why can't they ask me what I think? What will happen if I can't treat my child three times a day? If you reflect on these questions you will see that you are not the only one who is reasoning or thinking or making decisions. If you are trying to provide client-centred care, or if that is what your client/patient is expecting or demanding, what does it mean for your communication? It means recognising that you may know more about your profession and what it can offer than the patient and their family/carers, but they know more about their body or their child (etc.) than you do. It means that sometimes you need to teach people or provide them with enough information for them to be actively involved in decision making. It means talking *with* patients, making decisions *with* them, and working *with* them to achieve the goals you both agree on for their wellbeing. This collaboration obviously varies in level and style depending on the age, mental capacity, and wishes of your client. But remember that communication is a two-way activity. It is not just you telling people what you have decided is best for them and expecting them to comply.

27.1 Communicating reasoning

HANDY HINT

- Understand the purpose of your communication. What reasoning are you trying to convey or share?
- Recognise the needs and background of your audience and adjust your communication accordingly.
- Think about the context (e.g. formal, informal, emergency, scholarly debate) and tailor your communication to this context.
- Remember, communication is all about human interaction.

Being credible: Articulating and providing evidence for your reasoning

Apart from using a language style that is appropriate for your audience, being credible requires giving an explanation of the rationale of your reasoning. This is a challenging task for several reasons.

First, reasoning can happen rapidly, at a rather subconscious level. Our minds process many pieces of information quickly, and we often do not articulate all the connections we make in thinking (such as which of the many factors in the clinical situation make it preferable to choose one treatment option over another). In the classroom and during clinical education, students are encouraged to slow down and 'unbundle' their thinking so that they can explain the decisions they are making and the basis for these decisions. When they do this, students are often surprised at how much they actually know about their professional role and the rationales for proposed actions. They can also find out how much they still need to learn about people, their conditions, and their health-care needs.

Second, you need to provide evidence to justify your clinical decisions. Evidence for practice can be equated to knowledge. There are many ways of generating knowledge, ways that include but are not limited to research. It is important to understand that credible knowledge, or evidence for practice, can be derived from practice as well as from research. In a recent publication, Higgs et al. (2004, p. ix) argued that 'knowing how practice knowledge is created, used and developed (further) should become an explicit dimension of the core, the regularity and the expectation of professional practice'.

Evidence includes:

- professional craft knowledge, or tested knowledge arising from practice experience (e.g. knowledge of the effectiveness of treatment strategies)
- propositional knowledge (knowledge from both quantitative and qualitative research into the effectiveness of clinical interventions); systematic reviews of the research literature can help you to collate and critique research-based evidence of best practice
- theoretical knowledge that provides a rationale for treatments or actions
- applied science knowledge (e.g. how the body works, how people interact, how cultural influences affect behaviour)
- data gained from interaction with the client (e.g. pain levels, needs and preferences, capacity to participate in treatment, fears and concerns).

All these forms of evidence can be used in clinical reasoning to make decisions that facilitate best practice for the patient or client in the particular situation.

HANDY HINT ☞ **27.2 Improving your clinical decision making**

- Spend some time thinking about how you make clinical decisions.
- Listen to how experienced practitioners justify and explain their decisions.
- Practise explaining your decisions with your peers and discussing the knowledge you are using to justify your decisions. Challenge each other to provide credible rationales. For example, ask 'How do you know that this professional craft knowledge is true?' and 'How credible is that theory as the basis for your treatment decisions?'

Conclusion

To analyse how well you communicate your reasoning, think through the following matters:

- What approach do you take to reasoning (hypothetico–deductive, narrative, etc.)?
- What ethical issues do you face in your clinical practice? How do you deal with these ethical issues?
- What do you think is important to say when talking to patients/clients or colleagues about your clinical or professional decisions?
- What difference does it make if you are talking to adults or to children, to patients or to clients in community settings, to patients or to their carers?

References

Elstein, A. S., Shulman, L. S. & Sprafka, S. A. 1978, *Medical Problem Solving: An Analysis of Clinical Reasoning*, Harvard University Press, Cambridge, Massachusetts.

Elstein, A. S., Shulman, L. S. & Sprafka, S. A. 1990, 'Medical problem solving: A ten year retrospective', *Evaluation and the Health Professions*, vol. 13, pp. 5–36.

Fleming, M. H. 1991, 'The therapist with the three track mind', *American Journal of Occupational Therapy*, vol. 45, pp. 1007–14.

Fonteyn, M. E. 1995, 'Clinical reasoning in nursing', in *Clinical Reasoning in the Health Professions*, eds J. Higgs & M. Jones, Butterworth-Heinemann, Oxford, pp. 60–71.

Groen, G. J. & Patel, V. L. 1985, 'Medical problem-solving: Some questionable assumptions', *Medical Education*, vol. 19, pp. 95–100.

Higgs, J. 2003, 'Do you reason like a (health) professional?', in *Becoming an Advanced Healthcare Practitioner*, eds G. Brown, S. Esdaile & S. Ryan, Butterworth Heinemann, Edinburgh, pp. 145–60.

Higgs, J. & Jones, M. (eds) 2000, *Clinical Reasoning in the Health Professions*, 2nd edn, Butterworth-Heinemann, Oxford.

Higgs, J., Richardson, B. & Abrandt Dahlgren, M. 2004, 'Preface', in *Developing Practice Knowledge for Health Professionals*, eds J. Higgs, B. Richardson & M. Abrandt Dahlgren, Butterworth-Heinemann, Oxford, p. ix.

Jones, M. A. 1992, 'Clinical reasoning in manual therapy', *Physical Therapy*, vol. 72, pp. 875–84.

Jones, M., Jensen, G. & Rothstein, J. 1995, 'Clinical reasoning in physiotherapy', in *Clinical Reasoning in the Health Professions*, eds J. Higgs & M. Jones, Butterworth-Heinemann, Oxford, pp. 72–87.

Schmidt, H. G., Norman, G. R. & Boshuizen, H. P. A. 1990, 'A cognitive perspective on medical expertise: Theory and implications', *Academic Medicine*, vol. 65, pp. 611–21.

WORKING AS A MEMBER OF A COMMUNITY HEALTH TEAM

Linda Portsmouth

KEY TOPICS

→ Community-based client care teams

→ Multidisciplinary and interdisciplinary teams

→ Health promotion teams

→ Communicating in teams

Introduction

Students and graduates in the health and social sciences often work in community health teams. This chapter deals with the two main types of health teams that work in the community: (a) teams that provide client care and (b) health promotion teams that aim to prevent health problems. Throughout the chapter the term 'client' is used to refer to both clients and patients. Cooperation and collaboration among team members and between the team and the community are explored. (The teamwork and communication skills required within teams are discussed in Chapters 23 and 24.)

The team approach to health is most useful when complex issues need to be managed using the perspectives of health and social science professionals with different knowledge and skills to gain a satisfactory resolution (Heinemann 2002). It is important to consider patterns of cooperation and collaboration between the different practitioners in a team, as a well-functioning team provides a better health service.

Community-based client care teams

Community-based client care teams are usually employed by a health or disability organisation. They can be large, consisting of people from many different health professions, such as Aboriginal health workers, audiologists, dentists, dieticians, disability care workers, doctors, nurses, occupational therapists, pharmacists, physiotherapists, podiatrists, psychologists, social workers, speech pathologists, teachers, teaching assistants, volunteers, welfare workers, and youth workers.

These teams may:

- help people with a short-term disability or health condition until the problem no longer requires management (e.g. palliative care or wound care)
- provide ongoing assistance to people with a chronic health condition or a long-term or permanent disability (e.g. a mental health disorder or arthritis)
- monitor groups within the community to ensure their continued health, and intervene or refer on for treatment when they detect a problem (e.g. child health clinics and school dental programs).

These teams provide direct assessment, treatment, and follow-up services, usually in environments where the clients spend a fair amount of time (for example, home, workplace, child care centre, school, or recreation centre). Teams are able to share information and skills with the people who surround their clients on a daily basis, such as families, friends, employers, teachers, and carers. This helps to improve the health and functioning of clients within supportive environments. The level of improvement of clients and their ability to function within their community are reviewed regularly.

These teams may be based in government-funded community health centres or services, schools for children with special needs, disability service organisations (e.g. the Cerebral Palsy Association), or non-government health organisations (e.g. the AIDS Council). The team members might see clients in their office or treatment room, or might visit clients at their home, workplace, or school. Some teams are based in a hospital or an office building, with members travelling from location to location by car. Many team members working with people with disabilities choose to observe their clients in a number of environments and at different times of the day, to build up a comprehensive picture of how well the clients are performing in different areas of their lives. Team members can even be based in different locations but work together with the same clients.

Differences in communication between hospital-based and community-based teams

The major differences in communication between hospital-based teams and community-based teams are as follows:

- Community-based teams usually have a flatter management structure, giving team members more autonomy. This leads to a communication style that is more equal and multidirectional and to problem solving by consensus.
- Communication with clients and their families can be more effective when they are seen in their home, workplace, or school. Community-based teams do not have to imagine

what is being described about the client's life outside of the hospital ward. They can see it, discuss it, and solve problems directly. Clients and their families and carers also feel more confident and are more honest when they are in their own territory.

- Because members of community-based teams have less direct contact with each other, they need to prepare for and make the most of their face-to-face interactions. They also need to be flexible enough to communicate with each other via telephone, email, and written reports.
- Members of community-based teams often have less direct contact with their supervisors. They need to be self-reliant but also able to recognise when they should seek support and advice.
- Hospital-based teams often work under the leadership of a doctor, whereas community-based teams usually do not. If a community-based team does not have a doctor as a member, the medical advice it can give will be limited. Many community-based teams liaise with their clients' general practitioners, often by telephone or email if the general practitioner cannot easily attend meetings.

Multidisciplinary and interdisciplinary teams

The terms 'multidisciplinary team' and 'interdisciplinary team' are often used interchangeably to describe teams composed of people from different professional disciplines. Actually these terms define the ends of a continuum of teamwork styles. According to Heinemann (2002), *multidisciplinary* teams have members who work side by side but within their own professional disciplines; they may communicate well with each other but they do not collaborate directly in client management. *Interdisciplinary* teams, by contrast, integrate their functions and work collaboratively to achieve team goals.

Community-based teams may exist anywhere on the continuum from multidisciplinary to interdisciplinary. Consider the three hypothetical teams in Case Study 28.1. These teams all provide care to pre-school children with developmental delays. They function in ways that place them at different points on the continuum. Each team consists of an audiologist, a doctor, an occupational therapist, a physiotherapist, a psychologist, a social worker, and a speech pathologist.

The ability of a group to work as a highly efficient interdisciplinary team does not necessarily come easily and naturally. Potential barriers to full interdependence in a team include staff turnover and an employing organisation that does not support the development of interdependence. According to Heinemann and Zeiss (2002), teams take time and may need training to develop interdependence, as they need to learn:

- where their roles are unique
- where their roles overlap
- to take each other's roles and points of view seriously
- to recognise which clients would benefit from an interdependent approach and which ones need only one member of the team to see them.

An effective collaborative team communicates well and decides as a group how the team will function. Team performance can be affected if members have not clearly delineated their roles, and 'turf battles' may result if members compete with each other (Heinemann 2002). Team performance can have an enormous impact on each team member's job satisfaction and on the service provided to the team's clients. The concept of interdependence can also be applied to working relations between teams and organisations within the community.

Multidisciplinary and interdisciplinary teams providing services to pre-school children with intellectual disabilities

Team A—a multidisciplinary team

Robert, a 2-year-old boy with Down syndrome, is referred to the team. He is assessed by every member of the team individually and at a separate time. Robert's mother and father, Carl and Rebecca, thus needed to attend seven appointments in the community clinic over 2 weeks. They are asked many of the same questions at each appointment. Carl and Rebecca find this very stressful. It is difficult for them to get time off work and they are confused about the different information and advice they are given. They haven't found anyone who can answer all of their questions and have to work out what questions will be best answered by which team members. Robert gets bored during the repetitive assessment sessions and stops performing at his best. Rebecca becomes anxious that some of the health professionals are not seeing the real Robert.

After all the assessments are complete, the team members meet to discuss what they have found. It is decided that Robert is in good health and has hearing within normal limits, and that the family is coping well and is in no particular difficulty. The psychologist finds that Robert has a moderate intellectual delay. The doctor, social worker, and psychologist decide to review his progress after 6 months. The physiotherapist, occupational therapist, and speech pathologist also find a moderate delay and decide to offer regular appointments so that they can give Carl and Rebecca ideas for home activities to help Robert develop his gross motor, fine motor, play, and communication skills. They each draw up a plan of intervention and see him individually, in rooms at the clinic, for 6 months. They each visit Robert's child care centre to give the child care workers ideas on how to help him to develop his skills. After the 6 months is up, the team members individually review his progress and meet to discuss their findings. Carl and Rebecca are invited to this meeting.

Team B—a more interdisciplinary, interdependent team

Kara, a 3-year-old with a developmental delay, is assessed during two visits at home—one from the psychologist and speech pathologist and one from the physiotherapist and occupational therapist. Kara's parents, John and Michelle, are asked only a few of the same questions twice. The team members pool their assessment results, noting that the GP has found Kara to be in good health before referral to the team, and then arrange for Kara to see the audiologist for a hearing test. The whole team meets with the parents to set Kara's priorities. Kara attends fortnightly sessions with the occupational therapist and speech pathologist that incorporate some ideas from the physiotherapist and psychologist. The sessions combine activities that promote gross motor skills, fine motor skills, play skills, and the communication that arises naturally during these activities. John and Michelle participate and encourage Kara to do similar activities with them at home. After a few weeks, Kara joins a series of weekly group sessions with three other children of similar age and needs. She enjoys being with the other children and John and Michelle gain much from their interaction with the other parents. The occupational therapist and physiotherapist run these groups and incorporate ideas provided by the speech pathologist for encouraging communication.

Team C—an interdependent interdisciplinary team

Cooper is a 2-year-old boy with a developmental delay. The team appoints one of its members to be the family's case coordinator. This is normally the member who they predict, based on the referral information, would be the main person (or one of the main people) involved with Cooper on an ongoing basis. The case coordinator in this case is the occupational therapist. She visits Cooper and his mother, Charlene, to carry out an initial assessment, asking one set of questions once. The answers are shared with the rest of the team later. The case coordinator is an experienced professional who has learned a great deal from the other members of the team, both informally and during formal training sessions. She is able to answer most of Charlene's questions and will get back to her with any answers that needed to be checked with other team members. The case coordinator meets with the social worker to ask for some information that Charlene requires.

The case coordinator and Charlene then identify priorities and decide on further assessment. Cooper visits the audiologist to have his hearing assessed. He is found to have a hearing problem and is referred to the ear, nose, and throat specialist. The physiotherapist and speech pathologist visit Cooper and Charlene at home at the same time as the case coordinator. They assess Cooper and provide some extra program ideas. The case coordinator and Charlene plan the intervention. This intervention involves different members of the team at different times, but is arranged and monitored by the case coordinator. Initially, the speech pathologist and the case coordinator visit weekly. They help Charlene to develop Cooper's communication and fine motor skills. As Cooper's communication skills improve and his hearing problem is resolved, the speech pathologist ceases to visit. The physiotherapist then begins to visit once a month. Charlene feels she understands and is in control of what is happening at all times.

Comments

Team A is a multidisciplinary team. The duplication of service it demonstrates, with every member working alone and undertaking all tasks from the viewpoint of his or her profession, is becoming rarer. Most community-based teams function like Team B, with a good level of cooperation and collaboration. A few teams are as interdependent as Team C. This level of interdependence is highly efficient and cost-effective. There is little duplication of service and, for the client, communicating with one team member is the same as communicating with every team member.

Communication with other community teams and organisations

Client care teams working within the community develop and maintain some level of communication and cooperation with individuals, teams, and organisations that influence the lives of their clients. This often happens on a client-by-client basis and it allows teams to provide better care and support to their clients. Case Study 28.2 is an example of the communication and cooperation between the service providers that assist a particular community client.

More formal cooperation and collaboration between community services is required when a number of clients are shared between service providers who overlap in function. A team may be formed consisting of representatives of all of the other teams, to facilitate communication and coordinate services. Since the 1970s there has been an increase in community-based health care in Australia and a growing interest in the most effective methods of coordinating service provision. Hammerton et al. (2002) found that some models/programs work by formalising existing communication, cooperation, and coordination, while others provide a 'one-stop

Communication and cooperation for a community client

A community-based rehabilitation team is assisting 75-year-old Louisa after a mild stroke. The team consists of a doctor, a nurse, an occupational therapist, a physiotherapist, a social worker, and a speech pathologist. Louisa lived alone before the stroke and managed her life well. She was healthy, except for having Type 2 diabetes. Louisa now has muscle weakness in her right leg, right arm, and right hand, and unclear speech. She has returned home but is not able to do all that she used to be able to, although slow recovery continues. She is close to her four adult children and two of her neighbours, who provide social support. Members of the team will get to know Louisa's children, neighbours, general practitioner, diabetes support nurse, home help, transport providers, and meals-on-wheels deliverers, and the people who arrange for Louisa to attend the weekly meeting of a local Italian seniors' club. Louisa's preferred language, the one she is most fluent in, is Italian, so the team will also liaise with interpreters.

These various individuals and teams have begun to communicate and coordinate their services. The social worker has arranged transport to the seniors' club and ensured that home help and meals on wheels do not come on the day that Louisa attends the club. Members of the rehabilitation team visit her at home and sometimes visit to see how she is functioning at the seniors' club. They give the club workers advice on how best to assist Louisa. Team members often visit when one or two of Louisa's children can be there to meet them and find out about their mother's progress. The team doctor communicates with Louisa's general practitioner and with the diabetes nurse who is checking Louisa's blood-sugar level regularly (now that she is unable to do this for herself).

shop', with a single phone number and location for the community to access. All of the projects they studied included a local steering committee composed of various health and community care service providers and consumer representatives to plan the programs and services. Teamwork across traditional health and community care boundaries was found to be a key ingredient in the success of these programs (Hammerton et al. 2002). The potential benefits of collaboration between community health services and non–government organisations (Jolley & Masters 2002) include:

- better use of resources
- better outcomes for clients, particularly those with complex needs
- a broader and more comprehensive range of services
- increased funding opportunities.

Community participation in health care

According to Bourke (2002, p. 37), 'there is abundant evidence that the most successful health projects, programs and policies not only involve consumer participation, but are initiated by the community'. Consumer participation in health services ensures that the services better meet community needs, but this participation takes time. It is difficult to gain input from representatives of all groups within the community and it requires health services to share power with consumers (Bourke 2002).

Community participation in health care can take many forms:
- consultation by government on proposed policies
- community surveys

- client feedback and evaluation
- complaints procedures
- representation on project steering committees
- membership of boards of management
- community panels for priority setting
- volunteer work
- user advocacy
- seeking information from consumer groups, such as support and self-help groups
- resident action groups and advocacy/pressure groups campaigning on public health issues, such as pollution and environmental protection
- community management (e.g. Aboriginal Community Controlled Health Organisations)
- community organisation and development (Baum 2002; Bourke 2002).

Client care teams may involve the community in their work through any of the above activities. Community development and advocacy activities related to public health issues, however, are usually employed by health promotion teams working to prevent or reduce health problems that affect the wider community. In some cultures, such as among Australian Aboriginal groups, it is more appropriate to consider community health rather than the health of individuals, as the culture itself views health as a more holistic concept that involves the 'social, emotional, and cultural well being of the whole community' (O'Connor-Fleming & Parker 2001, p. 210). This means that even if a team is targeting particular individuals it is preferable to involve the whole community.

Community education and awareness

Client care teams may also share their expertise with the community to heighten awareness of the problems faced by their clients. Some effective ways of doing this are by giving community talks, writing articles for newspapers and magazines, and participating in promotional work or events (e.g. World AIDS Day, National Diabetes Week, Schizophrenia Awareness Week, Safety in Schools Week, and Down Syndrome Awareness Week). See Chapter 15 for a discussion of how the team can effectively communicate about health to the community.

Health promotion teams

Community-based teams work to prevent disabilities and health problems from occurring in the first place. Their membership depends on the aims of the health promotion project and the organisation that is initiating the task. A road-crossing safety initiative for school children, for example, might involve representatives from parent groups, the government road authority, local government, the government education department, the independent schools association, the state drivers' association, the local cyclists' association, individual schools, and road safety lobby groups. The project might run focus groups with school children, so that the issue can be explored from the perspective of the target group. The project organisers will probably appoint health promotion professionals as project coordinator and project officers, to work solely on the project until it ends. They may hire communication specialists to help them develop educational and promotional materials as needed. They may also hire health promotion specialists to assist them to plan and evaluate their project.

Health promotion is not simply health education. It is a 'process of enabling individuals and communities to increase control over ... and ... improve their health' (WHO 1986, p.1). The framework of health promotion was formulated through the World Health Organization in 1986. The resulting Ottawa Charter (WHO 1986) calls on health professionals to prevent ill health by working with communities to:

- build healthy public policy by putting health on the agenda of policy-makers and increasing their awareness of the health implications of their decisions
- create living and working environments that are supportive of good health
- strengthen community action—that is, empower communities to control their own health by setting priorities, making decisions, and planning and implementing health strategies
- develop people's skills and knowledge about health
- reorient health services to move beyond the treatment of illness to its prevention.

The Jakarta Declaration advocated a partnership approach to health and stated that a combination of the above strategies is more effective than any single approach, and that community education and participation in decision making are essential: 'Health promotion is carried out by and with people, not on or to people' (WHO 1997, p. 5).

Health-promotion team members require highly developed communication skills, as they undertake a wide variety of educational, organisational, economic, and political activities, advocating for attitudinal, social, environmental, and behavioural changes that favour good health (Howat et al. 2003). The teams usually target specific groups within the community that are at risk of poor health or disability (e.g. from injury, asthma, heart disease, cancer, or HIV/AIDS). They aim to empower these groups and reduce any psychosocial or environmental risk factors (e.g. social isolation, low self-esteem, dangerous environment) and/or specific risk behaviours (e.g. smoking, physical inactivity, poor diet, speeding by drivers, excessive alcohol intake). Teams may thus be involved in tasks as diverse as lobbying politicians for a change in the law regarding tobacco marketing, advocating for safer school playgrounds or workplaces, planning a health education program with community representatives, developing a TV advertisement that illustrates the consequences to young male drivers of speeding, and running small support groups in which young women can learn how to negotiate safe sex. There are a number of frameworks that health promotion teams can utilise in choosing health promotion strategies (e.g. Maycock et al. 2001). There is a growing emphasis on working to influence social and environmental factors, as it has been discovered that behaviours do not change significantly when the factors that cause them remain (Baum 2002). It is difficult, for example, to give up smoking when you are under stress, are surrounded by people who are smoking, and can easily buy cigarettes in your workplace.

Communicating with key stakeholders

Health promotion teams need to communicate with 'key stakeholders'. These are the people and organisations in the community that:

- are members of the target group
- represent the target group (e.g. self-help groups, consumer groups, cultural groups)
- work with or care for members of the target group (e.g. community service providers, government service providers from a variety of sectors, such as health, welfare, transport, police, and public housing)
- have some influence over members of the target group (e.g. community TV, radio, or newspaper, educational institutions, role models)
- feel strongly and politically about the health issues (e.g. resident action groups, advocacy/pressure groups)
- have influence over the risk factors themselves (e.g. employers, businesses, local, state, and federal government politicians and authorities).

Many of the key stakeholders may already be members of the health promotion team. Key stakeholders need to be involved at all stages of the health promotion program: at initial conception, needs assessment, prioritisation, planning, implementation, and evaluation (including follow-up to see whether health changes were made). This is a time-consuming communication task, but it is necessary if the project is to provide the best health outcomes for the community. It is vital that community programs be based on what the community sees as its priorities, rather than on how health and social science professionals interpret health statistics. A program shaped by the various stakeholders in a community is far more likely to succeed in that community than one planned by a group of health professionals huddled around a meeting table, drinking lots of coffee, thinking about 'what's best for the community'.

'Community organisation' and 'community development'

These two terms are often used interchangeably, but have rather different meanings. *Community organisation* is the process by which community groups are helped to identify their problems, formulate goals, and develop and implement strategies for reaching these goals (Minkler 1997). The key concept here is that the health promotion team takes a major role in gaining community participation in every stage of the process. This is the most common form of community participation used in health promotion in Australia. Many health promotion organisations have an agenda that is firmly focused on a particular aspect of health and, although they need community participation, they are not really able to give total control of the process to a community that may not prioritise their health issue. The Heart Foundation, Kidney Foundation, and Cancer Foundation, for example, have a responsibility to work with communities in relation to the factors that lead to heart disease, kidney disease, and cancer, as opposed to other health areas, such as preventing falls by the elderly, motor vehicle accidents, or suicide.

Community development is the process of working on health issues with a 'bottom up' rather than a 'top down' approach. Communities are empowered to make decisions about their own health, developing their strength and confidence over time (Egger et al. 1999). Community development is thought to be most appropriate for lower socio-economic and disadvantaged communities (Egger et al. 1999; O'Connor-Fleming & Parker 2001), and its effectiveness can

HANDY HINT

☞ 28.1 Communicating with a community

Note: These principles are especially important when the health professionals in the team are not members of the community they are working with.

Taking a partnership approach

- Remember that you are an expert in your area of health but that your patients/clients are experts in their own health and their community. The person with the health problem or disability is the ultimate expert. The people who live with them are the next level of expertise. Involve them in everything you can.
- Seek out and get to know community opinion leaders and decision-makers, and involve them as much as you can. But also involve the least powerful people in the community.
- Respect everyone's opinion and try to find out why they hold those opinions. Try to see things from the community's point of view, and ask for feedback from the community on the accuracy of your views.

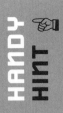

Learning about the community

- The more you know about a community, the better you will be able to communicate with the people. They will also feel respected and appreciate that you took the time to get to know them.
- Ask open questions that allow community members to answer as they wish to. Ask 'What do you want?' rather than 'Do you want this or that?'
- Try to find out as much as you can about the history of the health issue. What has been done before? What worked? What did not work? How did the community feel about it at the time? How do they feel about it now?
- Try not to have any preconceptions about what the community might want, need, or be experiencing.

Overcoming communication and partnership barriers

- Be consistent and honest. Trust will develop if you are predictable and your motives are clear.
- Lose your professional jargon. Learn how to say everything that you need to say in simple, straightforward language, especially if what you say is being translated into another language.
- If you are communicating with people who are not of your culture, religion, language, class, age, or gender, learn as much as you can about what you do not know. Work out, as best you can, what is appropriate for you to do and say, but be true to yourself. Don't pretend to be something that you are not.
- It may be better for community members, rather than health professionals, to communicate about health to their peers.
- Pass on skills and knowledge whenever you can, to whomever you can, in a way that respects the other person. Such generosity is rewarded in many ways.
- Give everybody continual feedback about what is happening. Team members need to know what each other are doing. Let team supervisors know about the team's communication with the community, and let the community know what the people in the health organisation are thinking. Convey what you learn from community groups to other sections of the community, unless what you have been told is confidential.
- Be flexible with your time-line for the project. Some communities may be able to communicate exactly what they need immediately; other communities will take more time.

most easily be seen in these communities (Webster 2002). This approach is important when the culture of the community is different from the culture of the health professionals. It has been used successfully in Aboriginal, refugee, and migrant communities. Community development has, however, also been a useful approach for less disadvantaged communities with health issues that affect all income groups, such as alcohol and drug use (Egger et al. 1999).

The health team and the community need to 'meet as equals and develop a dialogue based on trust' (Baum 2002, p. 369). The health promotion team's role is to be a coordinator, advocate, and catalyst (O'Connor-Fleming & Parker 2001, p. 185). Their task of facilitating action but being 'as unobtrusive as possible' may be difficult, due to conflicting employer and community agendas (Egger et al. 1999, p. 139). Health professionals can be caught between an employer who directs the team to do one thing and a community that wants to do something totally different. For this approach to work, health organisations and funding agencies need to give up some control to the community itself. If members of a non-Aboriginal organisation wish to work with Aboriginal people, for example, they need to know that they cannot fund a 6-month intervention program. The non-Aboriginal health workers will only just be beginning to gain the community's trust and establish tentative communication by the end of that time.

There is no one easy way to communicate and work with a community. Some general principles to guide health teams are given in Handy Hint 28.1.

Conclusion

Health teams, which have both client care and health promotion roles, can make profound positive changes to the lives and health of individuals and communities. Developing effective strategies for communication, cooperation, and collaboration, both within the team and with the community, is a vital part of achieving this goal.

References

Baum, F. 2002, *The New Public Health*, 2nd edn, Oxford University Press, Melbourne.

Bourke, L. 2002, 'Health consumer participation in coordinated care: A case study in the Goulburn Valley', *Australian Journal of Primary Health*, vol. 8, no. 1, pp. 37–44.

Egger, G., Spark, R., Lawson, J. & Donovan, R. 1999, *Health Promotion Strategies and Methods*, 2nd edn, McGraw-Hill, Sydney.

Hammerton, M., Sadler, P. & Cartwright, A. 2002, 'Teams that work', in *Communication for Health Care*, eds C. Berglund & D. Saltman, Oxford University Press, Melbourne, pp. 163–76.

Heinemann, G. D. 2002, 'Teams in health care settings', in *Team Performance in Health Care*, eds G. D. Heinemann & A. M. Zeiss, Kluwer Academic/Plenum Publishers, New York, pp. 3–18.

Heinemann, G. D. & Zeiss, A. M. 2002, 'A model of team performance', in *Team Performance in Health Care*, eds G. D. Heinemann & A. M. Zeiss, Kluwer Academic/Plenum Publishers, New York, pp. 29–42.

Howat, P., Maycock, B., Cross, D., Collins, J., Jackson, L., Burns, S. & James, R. 2003, 'Towards a unified definition of health promotion', *Health Promotion Journal of Australia*, vol. 14, no. 2, pp. 82–6.

Jolley, G. M. & Masters, S. 2002, 'Exploring the links between community health services and non-government organisations in two regions of South Australia', *Australian Journal of Primary Health*, vol. 8, no. 1, pp. 57–64.

Maycock, B., Howat, P. & Slevin, T. 2001, 'A decision making model for health promotion advocacy: The case for advocacy of drunk driving measures', *IUHPE Promotion and Education*, vol. 8, no. 2, pp. 59–64.

Minkler, M. 1997, *Community Organising and Community Building for Health*, Rutgers University Press, New Brunswick, New Jersey.

O'Connor-Fleming, M. L. & Parker, E. 2001, *Health Promotion*, 2nd edn, Allen and Unwin, Crows Nest, NSW.

Webster, I., 2002, 'Social inclusion and pubic health: The case for partnerships', *NSW Public Health Bulletin*, vol. 13, no. 6, pp. 133–6.

WHO—*see* World Health Organization.

World Health Organization 1986, *Ottawa Charter for Health Promotion*, WHO, Geneva <http://www.who.int/hpr/NPH/docs/ottawa_charter_hp.pdf> accessed 15 March 2004.

World Health Organization 1997, *The Jakarta Declaration on Leading Health Promotion into the 21st Century*, WHO, Geneva <http://www.who.int/hpr/NPH/docs/jakarta_declaration_en.pdf> accessed 15 March 2004.

Index

a and b referencing   65
academic honesty   5, 24, 26–7
academic writing *see* writing, academic
active listening   222
advocacy   232–3
angry people, communicating with   224
assessment, honesty in   26–7
assignments
    references   69–70
    writing   42–51
asynchronous communication   93–4
augumentative and alternative communication
        (AAC)   225–6

bad news, delivering   226–7
bibliographic catalogues   55–6
bibliographies   62–3
body language and culture   241

carers   219–20, 221–2
case conferences   120–5
case presentations   121–5
charts and clinical reports   110–11
chat rooms   96
citation index   57–8
citations   67
client care teams, community-based   261–6
client education   146–7
client records   110
clients
    and assertive communication   224
    and collusion   228
    strategies for effective communication   221–2
    talking with   219–20
clinical reasoning   254–8
clinical reports
    ethical and legal issues   113–15
    formats   108–13
    purposes of   106
    tips and strategies for   115–18
    types   107–8
    writing effective   115
clinical settings and ethics   27–8
colleagues
    strategies for effective communication   221–2
    talking with   219–20
collusion with clients   228

communication
    with angry people   224
    assertive   224, 249–51
    asynchronous   93–4
    challenging situations   223–8
    clinical reasoning   254–8
    confronting   249–51
    definition   4
    distance/flexible   96
    effective   12, 221–2
    electronic   90–8
    ethical   22–8
    health   138–50
    hospital-based teams   261–2
    importance of   4
    intercultural   239–45
    issues in   4–6, 223–8
    with key stakeholders   267–8
    miscommunication   242–3
    oral   10, 220–1
    with people who have trouble communicating
        224–6
    person-centred   10–11
    with a person with a disability   227
    problem-based learning classes   99–104
    process   7–9
    skills   10–11
    subjects outside your area of expertise   227–8
    synchronous   93–4, 95–6
    transactional model   9
    types of   6–7
    understanding   10
    with upset people   224
    verbal   10
    written   10
community-based client care teams   261–6
community development   268–70
community education and awareness   266
community health proposals   126–35
    budget proposal   130–1
    community profile   128–9
    example of successful   132–5
    making an argument   127–31
    needs assessment   129–30
    structure   127
    writing   127, 131–2
community organisation   268–70

community participation in health care 265–6
conferences 195
confidentiality 115, 228
consultative advice 231–2
copyright 24–5
counselling 146–7
credibility 6
cultural appropriateness 6
cultural competence 11
culture
    and body language 241
    and communication 239–45

database, organising your reference 68–9
databases 55–6
desktop conferencing 97
diagnostic reports 108–9
discharge reports 111
distance/flexible communication 96
document, planning the style of your 156–60
drafting 118
duty of care 114, 232

electronic communication 90–9
electronic messages 94–5
electronic reference-management systems 67–8
electronic reference-storage systems 71
email 97
essays, writing 42–51
    analysing the topic 42–3
    body 44
    conclusion 44
    formatting for headings 46
    headings, use of 45
    illustrative material 48
    images on the Internet 48
    introduction 44
    plan 44–5
    reference material 46–8
    sketch diagram 45
    structure 43–5
    supporting your case 45–8
    Web information, reliability of 47
    see also writing
et al. 66
ethical communication 22–8
ethical group work 25–6
ethical issues and clinical reports 113–15
ethical research work 25
ethics 5, 23–4
exams 26–7

feedback 247–53
    characteristics of effective, constructive 248,
        250
    dimensions 248
    factors influencing 251–3
    purposes of 248
    reasons for 249–51

fieldwork settings and ethics 27–8
flexible learning 90–9
fonts 156–7

grammar 49–50
graphics and tables 161–7
graphics, labelling 167
group(s)
    and advocacy 232–4
    balancing process 206–8
    and consultative advice 231–2
    facilitating task completion 212–13
    leaders 211–12
    and mediation 234–6
    meetings 214–16
    member, roles of 208–10
    and negotiation 236–8
    problem solving 213–14
    understanding 206

hard-copy reference-management systems 71–2
health behaviour change 140–6
health care, community participation 265–6
health communication
    channels 141–5
    definition 138–9
    face-to-face client education 146–7
    mass media 147–50
    process 138, 139–40
health promotion teams 266–70
honesty see academic honesty; ethics
hospital-based teams 261–2
humanity 4–5

ibid. 66
illustrative material 48
individuals and mediation 234–6
information
    locating 53–7
    management 114
    ownership 115
    systematically recording, storing, and
        retrieving 58–9
    see also literature-searching
informed consent 114–15
intellectual property 24
interactive text communication 10
intercultural communication 239–45
intercultural competence 240
interdisciplinary teams 262–4
Internet 56–7
interpreters 244–5

journal papers 73–9
    choosing the right journal 74–5
    designing the paper 76–7
    editing and revising 77
    preparation for submission 77–8
    responding to reviewers 78

writing plan   75
writing with colleagues   75–6

leadership
    group   211–12
    style and control   210
learning   19–20
    flexible   90–9
legal issues and clinical reports   113–15
libraries   53–4
listening, active   222
literature-searching
    effective   53
    skills   52–3
    using a citation index   57–8
    see also information

mass media health communication   147–50
mediation   234–6
medico-legal reports   112–13
meetings   214–16
miscommunication   242–3
multicultural countries   240
multidisciplinary teams   262–4
multimedia environment   92–3

negotiation
    achieving optimal outcomes   236–8
    one-to-one   237

online environment   92–3
op cit.   66
oral communication   10
    principles of effective   220–1
organisational skills   19
outline view   160
ownership of information   115

page numbers   66
paragraphing   49
paraphrasing   66
person-centred communication   10–11
pictures, use of   166
plagiarism   25
posters   169–75
    creating on a computer   170
    layout and text   170–3
    legibility, font, and colour   173–5
    transporting   170
    using images   175
PowerPoint presentations   184–93, 197
    animation   192
    clip art   188
    editing   192
    good presentations   185
    hyperlinks   191–2
    notes   188
    photos, tables, and graphs   188–91
    planning   185–6

practising your presentation   193
    simple, creating a   186–92
    slides and text   188
    templates   187–8
primary source   61–2
printers and software   158
problem-based learning classes   99–104
problem solving in groups   213–14
professional honesty   5
professionalism   6, 11, 12, 27–8
progress notes and clinical reports   110
proofreading   87, 118
punctuation   49–50

quotations   65

records, keeping   58
reference database, organising your   68–9
reference lists   62–3
    developing and storing your own   67
reference-management systems
    electronic   67–8
    hard-copy   71–2
reference material for essays   46–8
reference-storage systems, electronic   71
referencing
    a and b   65–6
    citations   67
    conventions   62
    describing your own work   66–7
    in drafts   65
    et al.   66
    guidelines   62
    Harvard system   63, 64
    ibid.   66
    op cit.   66
    page numbers   66
    paraphrasing   6
    resources on   63
    and sources   61–2
    strategies   65–7
    style   62
    systems, major   63
    tools   65–6
references
    assignment, thesis, or paper   69–70
    formatting for a writing task   70–1
    managing   71
    principles of storing   68
referrals   112
report writing   115–18
research paradigms   82
research work, ethical   25
resources, effective storage and retrieval   58–9

sans-serif fonts   156–7
Sciences Citation Index (SCI)   58
searching see literature-searching
secondary sources   62

self-evaluation 6
self-monitoring 11
self-reflection 6
sentences, writing short 49
serif fonts 156–7
shortcut keys 158
Social Sciences Citation Index (SSCI) 58
sources
    primary and secondary 61–2
    and referencing 61–2
speaking at conferences 195
speaking to an audience you know well 178–9
spelling 50
standards 5
study
    skills 15–20
    space 19
    time 16–19
synchronous communication 93–4, 95–6

table of contents 160
tables
    and graphics 161–7
    with numerical data 165
    with word data 164–5
talking
    adapting your style 222–3
    with colleagues, patients, clients, and carers
        219–20
talks at conferences 194–201
    abstracts 195–6
    audio-visual arrangements 197
    audio-visual support 199–200
    body of the talk 199
    conclusion 199
    confidence 200
    papers grouped with yours 197
    preliminary preparation 196–7
    presentation effectiveness 197–9
    question time 201
    rehearsing 200
    target audience 196
    time allocation 196
    venue 197
talks in class 176–82
    audience attention, maintaining 180
    different styles 177
    introducing, discussing, and concluding
        179–82
    question time 182
    reasons to give 176–7
    speaking to an audience 178–9
    visual aids 180–1
task assessment 16
teams
    community-based client care 261–6
    health promotion 266–70
    multidisciplinary and interdisciplinary 262–4

telephone conferencing 96–7
templates 159–60
text style and formatting 155–60
texts, recommended 54–5
thesis writing 80–8
    critique 86
    layout and presentation 84
    preparation 85–6
    proofing/printing 87
    reflection 86
    structure 82–3
    style 83–5, 156–60
    and supervisors 87
    technical aspects 85
    what makes a good thesis 81–2
    writing phase 86
    the writing task 85–7
thesis references 69–70
time assessment 16–18
time management 17–18, 19
timetables 18–19
topic analysis 42–3

universities and ethics 23–4
upset people, communicating with 224

verbal communication 10
videoconferencing 97
visual aids, advantages and disadvantages 180–1
voicemail 96

Web information, reliability 47
word data with tables 164–5
word limits for essays 50–1
Word styles 158–9
writing
    academic, characteristics of 30
    assignments 42–51
    effect of culture 34
    free 45
    grammar 49–50
    paragraphing 49
    presentation 50–1
    problems 31–2
    process 34–7
    punctuation 49–50
    report 115–18
    short sentences 49
    skills, basic 33
    spelling 50
    task, formatting references 70–1
    technical aspects of 38–41
    types and formats 30–2
    well 49–51
    word limits 50–1
    see also essay writing; journal papers; thesis
        writing
written communication 10